Test Bank
to Accompany

ABNORMAL PSYCHOLOGY:
A DISCOVERY APPROACH

by
Steven Schwartz

Anita Rosenfield
The DeVry Institute of Technology
Chaffey College

Mayfield Publishing Company
Mountain View, California
London • Toronto

International Standard Book Number 0-7674-1423-3

Manufactured in the United States of America
10   9   8   7   6   5   4   3   2

Mayfield Publishing Company
1280 Villa Street
Mountain View, California 94041
(650) 960-3222

CONTENTS

PREFACE

Why a test bank? The obvious answer is, "to make the professor's life easier!" Although the "uninitiated" may think our lives consist merely of preparing and giving classroom lectures, we are all aware that the great bulk of our work rests in out-of-class tasks. (For me, the most time-consuming is grading papers.) Thus, writing exams can become extremely burdensome, especially if you are like me and give three midterms and a comprehensive final each term. In fact, I know many instructors who give a quiz every week. And, as much as many of us may wish this weren't the case, tests remain one of the primary methods we have for assessing our students' performance.

Personally, I use tests not only to assess student performance, but also as a teaching tool, a way to reinforce information and encourage students to think about the material. Consequently, the questions I write (both in this test bank and for my other classes) are designed with both goals in mind: to assess and to educate.

With respect to the latter goal, I have heard it said that "good" test questions make students think and require them to choose among several potentially tempting options. I try to keep that admonition in mind while writing test items, yet it makes me think about Lashley's rats, who, having to choose between two stimuli that were so similar as to be almost indistinguishable, developed experimental neurosis. I try to avoid that as much as possible. Further, to keep students from becoming so discouraged that they give up in frustration, I believe they need some questions that allow them to take a breather and say to themselves, "Wow! Got that one. I guess I do know something!" So, scattered throughout are some questions that may seem obvious. (It is not only faculty who need their load lightened.) In the end, however, it is up to instructors to choose the questions that they believe are most appropriate to meet their teaching goals.

The test bank consists of at least 60 multiple-choice questions (usually more), 20 true-false questions, 15 short-answer questions, and 5 essay questions. Answers are provided for all of the multiple-choice and true-false questions, they are written out in full for the short-answer questions, and the basic ideas are provided for the essay questions. Following each question except the essay questions is the page number and topic where the information can be found.

There are almost no dates and few numbers in these questions. That is my personal choice because I find these hard to remember—as a consequence, I rarely ask my students to remember them. Aside from that intended omission, the questions include factual, conceptual, and applied information and range from relatively simple to more complex and challenging.

Each of us, of course, has a different teaching style, just as our students have different learning styles. Some instructors prefer to remain as close to the text as possible; others prefer to bring in additional information, whether from their own clinical experience, their research, or other readings. The more we diverge from the text, the more likely we are to want to write some of our own questions to reflect our lectures. (I've had students who get upset with me because I test them on material from a classroom lecture that wasn't in the book—but it does tend to keep them coming to class!) If, like me, that is your style, of course you will need to create those questions yourself to pepper throughout your exams. The purpose of this test bank is to make your life easier, so you do not have to write the whole term's worth of exams and you have a wide choice of questions to reflect the information you wish your students to internalize.

I hope you find this test bank useful and that it does, indeed, help lighten your out-of-classroom load so that you can enjoy your time in the classroom with your students as much as I enjoy my classroom time with mine. Happy teaching.

Anita Rosenfield

CHAPTER 1
THE DEATH OF DANIELLE WOOD

MULTIPLE-CHOICE QUESTIONS

1. The opening paragraph of Chapter 1 indicates that the parents of these college students believe that
   *a. because things seem not to have changed since they were students at this college, the campus is a safe place for their children.
   b. security has increased since they were students at this college, so it must be a safe place for their children.
   c. on college campuses, students are assured of a safe and stimulating environment.
   d. there have been radical changes since they were students at this college, causing them to be alarmed for their children.

   Page: 2   Topic: The Death of Danielle Wood

2. In the newspaper article about Danielle's death, all of the following suggest that she committed suicide EXCEPT:
   a. she had a history of suicide attempts.
   *b. she left a suicide note.
   c. she had a terrible childhood and a stormy relationship.
   d. she had recently missed making the Olympic team.

   Pages: 2–3   Topic: Document 1.1 Newspaper Report of Danielle's Death

3. Based on the newspaper article reporting Danielle's death, it is possible that, instead of being suicide, her death was due to
   a. an infection contracted during her recent stay at the student health services hospital.
   b. a covered-up rape-homicide.
   *c. an overdose of steroids and amphetamines.
   d. heart failure caused by overexertion in swimming.

   Page: 3   Topic: Document 1.1 Newspaper Report of Danielle's Death

4. The social work report prepared after Danielle's first suicide attempt stated that her suicide gesture was
   a. a desperate attempt to end a life of abuse.
   b. an accidental drug overdose.
   c. nearly successful.
   *d. a way of getting attention and controlling her boyfriend.

   Page: 6   Topic: Document 1.2 Social Work Report Prepared After Danielle's Suicide Attempt

5. According to Danielle's psychological assessment, which test was given as an intellectual assessment?
   *a. Wechsler Adult Intelligence Scale–Third Edition (WAIS-III)
   b. Minnesota Multiphasic Personality Inventory (MMPI-2)
   c. Thematic Apperception Test (TAT)
   d. Rorschach Inkblot Test

   Page: 6   Topic: Document 1.3 Psychological Assessment Prepared Following Danielle's Previous Suicide Attempt

1

6. An indicator of Danielle's depression on the WAIS-III was
   a. her responses to questions concerning her mood.
   *b. the slowness of her responses on performance tasks.
   c. her reluctance to answer many of the questions.
   d. a comparison of her low score on that test with her scholastic record.

   Page: 7   Topic: Document 1.3 Psychological Assessment Prepared Following Danielle's Previous Suicide Attempt

7. Danielle's responses on the MMPI-2 indicated all of the following EXCEPT that she
   a. felt apathetic and indifferent to her usual activities.
   b. believed that her life was no longer under her control.
   *c. had considerable self-dislike and self-blame.
   d. was experiencing a loss of energy and an inability to feel pleasure.

   Page: 7   Topic: Document 1.3 Psychological Assessment Prepared Following Danielle's Previous Suicide Attempt

8. The test that demonstrated Danielle's preoccupation with success and her fear of failure was the
   a. Minnesota Multiphasic Personality Inventory (MMPI-2).
   b. Beck Depression Inventory (BDI).
   c. Wechsler Adult Intelligence Scale–Third Edition (WAIS-III).
   *d. Thematic Apperception Test (TAT).

   Page: 7   Topic: Document 1.3 Psychological Assessment Prepared Following Danielle's Previous Suicide Attempt

9. President Reynolds tells the students about a new program that is being initiated, which was inspired by Danielle's suicide. This program includes all of the following EXCEPT
   *a. psychological evaluations of all students entering the college for the first time.
   b. a pamphlet containing the warning signs of suicide.
   c. special classes for dormitory resident advisers to teach them to recognize the warning signs of suicide.
   d. a peer education program in which resident advisers and other students trained in stress management will talk to groups of students.

   Page: 10   Topic: The Death of Danielle Wood

10. The text notes that answers to questions about abnormal psychology (e.g., "What is abnormal behavior?" "What causes it?") have
   a. remained relatively constant for centuries.
   *b. changed as social attitudes evolved.
   c. changed in some cultures over time but have remained relatively constant in the United States.
   d. remained relatively constant in nonindustrial societies but have changed dramatically in technologically advanced cultures.

   Page: 11   Topic: How Did Danielle Die?

11. The text warns that it is natural to identify with the cases in the text. It suggests the best way to handle this is to
   a. understand that we all have the potential to develop the disorders discussed.
   b. recognize how different we are from the individuals discussed in the case studies.
   *c. examine each case in depth to understand that we are not identical to the person described.
   d. avoid the temptation to compare our own situations with those in the case studies.

   Page: 11   Topic: How Did Danielle Die?

12. In assessing the reasons given for Danielle's death, it becomes clear that
    a. they tend to cluster around the social forces in Danielle's life.
    b. the mental health professionals (the psychiatrist, the psychologist, and the social worker) most likely have the best explanations.
    c. genetics was undoubtedly the primary issue because, as Mrs. Wood pointed out, Danielle's father also took his own life.
    *d. biological, psychological, and social forces all played a part.

    Page: 11   Topic: Why Did Danielle Die?

13. Modern clinical psychologists refer to behavior as _____ because biological, psychological, and social forces all interact to determine our actions.
    *a. biopsychosocial
    b. physiopsychosocial
    c. sociological
    d. sociocultural

    Page: 11   Topic: Why Did Danielle Die?

14. The primary difference between a psychologist who holds a PhD and one who holds a PsyD is that the
    a. PhD requires more education.
    *b. PsyD requires intensive clinical training.
    c. PhD requires intensive clinical training.
    d. PsyD requires a more elaborate dissertation.

    Page: 12   Topic: Highlight 1.1 Who's Who in Mental Health?

15. All of the following are required of clinical psychologists in most states in the United States EXCEPT
    a. a doctoral degree.
    b. closely supervised internships.
    *c. sponsorship by a licensed therapist.
    d. passing a special examination to receive certification or licensure.

    Page: 12   Topic: Highlight 1.1 Who's Who in Mental Health?

16. The education for clinical psychologists places special emphasis on
    a. everyday problems.
    b. marriage counseling.
    c. developmental issues.
    *d. research techniques.

    Page: 12   Topic: Highlight 1.1 Who's Who in Mental Health?

17. Dr. Kahn is a psychiatrist. Which of the following degrees does she have?
    *a. MD
    b. PsyD
    c. PhD
    d. MSW

    Page: 12   Topic: Highlight 1.1 Who's Who in Mental Health?

18. Psychiatrists are most likely to view psychological problems as
    a. adjustment problems.
    *b. illnesses.
    c. stress related.
    d. arising from unconscious conflicts.

    Page: 12   Topic: Highlight 1.1 Who's Who in Mental Health?

19. The mental health professional most likely to view behavioral problems as the result of unconscious conflicts arising from early childhood experiences is the
   a. psychiatrist.
   b. psychologist.
   *c. psychoanalyst.
   d. psychiatric social worker.

   Page: 12   Topic: Highlight 1.1 Who's Who in Mental Health?

20. As an MSW, Li Cheong would primarily
   a. work in a hospital setting.
   b. be engaged in therapy with children.
   c. do administrative work with a team of mental health professionals.
   *d. focus on integrating people into their respective communities.

   Page: 12   Topic: Highlight 1.1 Who's Who in Mental Health?

21. Which mental health professional would most likely play a largely rehabilitative role?
   *a. occupational therapist
   b. psychiatric social worker
   c. psychologist
   d. counselor

   Page: 12   Topic: Highlight 1.1 Who's Who in Mental Health?

22. When Sigmund Freud said, "Biology is destiny," he meant that our
   a. genetic inheritance predisposes us to certain psychological traits.
   *b. personalities are strongly determined by whether we are male or female.
   c. biological traits have a stronger influence over us than our experiences.
   d. life course cannot be altered by environmental influences.

   Page: 11   Topic: Can Depression and Suicidal Behavior Be Inherited?

23. Twins who come from the same fertilized egg are referred to as _____ twins.
   a. fraternal
   b. dizygotic
   *c. monozygotic
   d. conjoined

   Page: 13   Can Depression and Suicidal Behavior Be Inherited?

24. Studies comparing monozygotic and dizygotic twins are particularly important because
   a. compared with other siblings or nonrelated children, it is easier to study twins' environments as they mature.
   b. twins are more likely than other children to share both genes and environment.
   c. they provide a natural laboratory for assessing what happens if one twin's genes are altered.
   *d. if behavior has a genetic origin, then the more closely related people are, the more similar we would expect their behavior to be.

   Page: 13   Topic: Can Depression and Suicidal Behavior Be Inherited?

25. The concordance rate for suicide among identical twins is approximately _____%.
   *a. 20
   b. 50
   c. 70
   d. 100

   Page: 13   Topic: Can Depression and Suicidal Behavior Be Inherited?

26. Which model of abnormal psychology would explain someone's committing suicide in terms of needing both a genetic predisposition and some precipitating stress?
    a. biological
    *b. diathesis-stress
    c. biopsychosocial
    d. psychodynamic

    Page: 14   Topic: Can Depression and Suicidal Behavior Be Inherited?

27. Drugs that can alleviate the symptoms of psychological disorders are called _____ drugs.
    a. placebo
    b. psychosomatic
    *c. psychotropic
    d. mood-elevating

    Page: 14   Topic: Did Danielle's Death Have a Physiological Origin?

28. Amphetamines are drugs that
    a. usually calm people down.
    b. improve physical performance.
    c. reduce psychotic symptoms (such as hallucinations).
    *d. after continued use may cause people to lose contact with reality.

    Page: 14   Topic: Did Danielle's Death Have a Physiological Origin?

29. The idea that psychological disorders can have physical causes dates back to
    *a. the ancient Greeks.
    b. biblical times.
    c. 19th-century Europe.
    d. the 1940s in the United States.

    Page: 14   Topic: Did Danielle's Death Have a Physiological Origin?

30. How do modern theories of abnormalities parallel those of ancient Greece?
    a. Both believe that drugs can alleviate abnormalities.
    *b. Both attribute depression and suicide to imbalances in brain chemistry.
    c. Both attribute depression and suicide to an excess of black bile.
    d. Both use the term *melancholer* as a synonym for depression.

    Page: 15   Topic: Did Danielle's Death Have a Physiological Origin?

31. Archeologists have found numerous ancient skulls with symmetrical holes that appear to have been intentionally drilled (that is, trephining). Most psychologists today believe that trephining was a
    a. result of warfare.
    b. treatment for removing splinters of bone and blood clots.
    *c. treatment for mental disorders.
    d. religious rite.

    Page: 16   Topic: Highlight 1.2 Why We Should Never Judge the Past by the Present

32. Our current belief that trephining was a treatment for mental disorders aimed at releasing evil demons from the brain demonstrates
    a. the result of rational and scientific research.
    b. how oral histories can become distorted over generations of transmission.
    c. an educated medical "guess" that provides a likely explanation.
    *d. the imposition of the standards of one civilization on another civilization.

    Page: 16   Topic: Highlight 1.2 Why We Should Never Judge the Past by the Present

33. The text relates stories (such as Foucault's "ship of fools") that demonstrate how psychological research can be easily biased by the acceptance of unsubstantiated or misinterpreted accounts of earlier events. These are examples of
    *a. presentism.
    b. cultural bias.
    c. cultural relativism.
    d. concordance.

    Page: 17 Topic: Highlight 1.2 Why We Should Never Judge the Past by the Present

34. Glenn, who was in the late stages of AIDS, was suffering from dementia. Which biogenic cause of abnormal behavior would most likely be contributing to Glenn's dementia?
    a. aberrant physiology
    *b. infectious illness
    c. damaged anatomy
    d. physical trauma

    Page: 15 Topic: Did Danielle's Death Have a Physiological Origin?

35. After assessing Mesmer's techniques for clearing blockages of "magnetic fluid," which led to a variety of ills, the French Royal Commission concluded that
    a. Mesmer had come up with a fascinating and useful technique.
    b. Mesmer's patients were frauds.
    *c. Mesmer's patients suffered from psychological problems that were eliminated by "suggestion."
    d. none of Mesmer's patients had been cured; instead, they were all defrauding the public.

    Page: 16 Topic: Mesmerism and the Birth of Modern Abnormal Psychology

36. As seen from Danielle's case in the text, people (particularly children) who are subjected to abuse and cannot stop it may develop learned helplessness. This, in turn, typically leads to all of the following EXCEPT
    a. depression.
    b. suicide.
    c. a belief that they cannot control their lives.
    *d. rebellious behavior.

    Page: 18 Topic: Possible Psychological Contributions to Danielle's Death

37. Jason has limited interactions with other people, and those he does have are unsatisfying. His depression is more difficult to treat than that of someone who has a circle of supportive friends. This illustrates
    *a. social isolation.
    b. learned helplessness.
    c. guilt.
    d. a sense of loss.

    Page: 18 Topic: Possible Psychological Contributions to Danielle's Death

38. Across Europe, from the 14th to the 16th centuries, a strange phenomenon occurred in which people threw off their clothing, danced wildly through the streets, foamed at the mouth, and babbled in strange tongues. The term derived from that behavior that is now used to describe the odd muscle movements that accompany some forms of brain disorder is
    a. tarantism.
    *b. St. Vitus' dance.
    c. presentism.
    d. whirling dervishism.

    Page: 18 Topic: Was Danielle's Death the Result of Social and Cultural Factors?

39. With regard to the relationship between psychological disorders and economics, as unemployment increases,
    a. the number of admissions to mental hospitals decreases.
    b. there is no change in the number of admissions to mental hospitals.
    *c. the number of admissions to mental hospitals increases.
    d. fewer people are admitted to mental hospitals, but more people with psychological disorders are seen among the homeless.

    Page: 19   Topic: Was Danielle's Death the Result of Social and Cultural Factors?

40. In the case of Danielle's suicide,
    a. it is likely that her father's suicide in some way caused hers.
    b. there is no way to know if her father's suicide caused hers.
    c. most likely her father's suicide was unrelated to hers.
    *d. Danielle and her father may both have been driven to suicide by some common factor, such as an inherited disposition.

    Page: 21   Topic: The Cause of Danielle's Death: What Can We Conclude?

41. A common malady in Malaysia until the implementation of the British judicial system was running amok. This involved
    *a. frenzied rampages that resulted in indiscriminate killings.
    b. running naked through the streets.
    c. total emotional withdrawal characterized by lack of speech and social interaction.
    d. major depression.

    Page: 20   Topic: Highlight 1.3 Running Amok

42. When considering abnormal behavior from the perspective that it differs from the norm, you are using a _____ viewpoint.
    a. mental health
    *b. statistical
    c. utilitarian
    d. social values

    Page: 21   Topic: Danielle's Behavior Was Unusual

43. The perspective on abnormality that uses a balancing of costs and benefits to determine if someone is "dangerous" (and thus requires hospitalization and observation) or "not dangerous" (and thus can be treated less intrusively) is the _____ approach.
    a. diathesis-stress
    b. utilitarian
    *c. statistical
    d. social values

    Page: 22   Topic: Danielle's Behavior Was Unusual

44. Aisha, a highly sensitive artist who agreed to participate in research on depression, was administered the Los Angeles Suicide Prevention Center Lethality Scale (Shneidman, Farberow, & Litman, 1970). She was shocked to learn that her score fell toward the upper range of the "indeterminate" area of overlap between suicidal and not-suicidal scores. Aisha had never considered taking her own life. Her score was a
    a. true-negative.
    b. true-positive.
    c. false-negative.
    *d. false-positive.

    Page: 23   Topic: Critical Thinking about Clinical Decisions 1.1: How Many Suicides Can We Afford to Prevent?

45. The notion of *parens patriae* assumes that people are
   *a. not always able to make appropriate decisions for themselves, so the government must step in to make decisions on their behalf.
   b. not always able to make appropriate decisions for themselves, so their families must step in to make decisions on their behalf.
   c. typically the best judge of their own needs and their own distress levels, and thus are best able to make decisions on their own behalf.
   d. best cared for by their parents if they cannot take care of themselves.

   Page: 24   Topic: Danielle's Behavior Produced Distress

46. When considering what constitutes abnormality, utilitarians look at
   a. the distress felt by the individual.
   *b. whether behavior causes harm to the individual or society (or both).
   c. how unusual the behavior is.
   d. whether the behavior falls within social norms.

   Page: 24   Topic: Danielle's Behavior Produced Distress

47. All of the following have been culturally respected (and often expected) ways to end one's life EXCEPT
   a. Bushido
   b. hara-kiri
   *c. amok
   d. suttee

   Page: 25   Topic: Danielle's Behavior Violated Social Values

48. The person whose research demonstrated that homosexuals are as well-adjusted as heterosexuals was
   a. Alfred Kinsey.
   b. William Masters.
   c. Virginia Johnson.
   *d. Evelyn Hooker.

   Page: 26   Topic: Critical Thinking about Clinical Decisions 1.2: Homosexuality and the Politics of Psychiatric Diagnosis

49. Brenda believes that people are plotting against her. Craig believes he receives daily messages from God. Both Brenda and Craig are suffering from
   *a. delusions.
   b. hallucinations.
   c. general paresis.
   d. brain damage.

   Page: 25   Topic: General Paresis and Mental Illness

50. Although the symptoms of general paresis appear to be a form of mental illness, in reality they are linked to the physical disease of
   a. tuberculosis.
   *b. syphilis.
   c. gonorrhea.
   d. herpes.

   Page: 25   Topic: General Paresis and Mental Illness

51. The analogy between medical and psychological disorders can be criticized on all of the following grounds EXCEPT
   a. illusory explanations.
   b. cultural biases.
   *c. scientific purposes.
   d. cultural biases.

   Page: 28   Topic: Differentiating Between Physical and Mental Disorders

52. A major difference between physical illnesses and psychological disorders is that
   a. the causes of physical illnesses are generally known.
   b. most physical illnesses are limited to specific geographic areas.
   c. most psychological disorders are universally recognized.
   *d. most psychological disorders are linked to certain cultures and times.

   Page: 25   Topic: Differentiating Between Physical and Mental Disorders

53. Zachary has been referred for a psychological assessment to determine whether he might be suicidal. Under normal conditions, we would expect the assessment to include all of the following EXCEPT
   *a. interviews with his parents.
   b. psychological testing.
   c. observations of Zachary's behavior.
   d. an in-depth interview with Zachary and a review of his records to develop a case history.

   Page: 29   Topic: Why Clinical Predictions Are Often Uncertain

54. The text notes that mental health professionals have difficulty predicting behavior for all of the following reasons EXCEPT:
   a. diagnoses do not suggest a specific etiology or treatment, nor do they lead to a specific prognosis.
   *b. due to the high rate of false-positive results on tests, such as the suicide lethality scale, mental health professionals are reluctant to make behavioral predictions.
   c. the main sources of clinical information is typically self-reports, which are notoriously unreliable.
   d. some of the tests that are given to assess psychological disorders have low predictive validity.

   Page: 29   Topic: Diagnosis

55. Oskamp's (1965) study of the relationship between the amount of information available and psychologists' confidence in the accuracy of their predictions suggests that
   a. the more information psychologists have, the better are their predictions.
   b. the more information psychologists have, the less reliable are their predictions.
   *c. psychologists are not always good judges of their own accuracy.
   d. whether a psychologist makes a good behavioral prediction depends on both the amount of information available and the particular diagnosis.

   Page: 30   Topic: Clinical versus Statistical Prediction

56. In comparison with Oskamp's (1965) findings concerning clinical predictions, Meehl (1954) believed that
   a. clinical predictions are more reliable than statistical predictions.
   b. clinical predictions are equally as reliable as statistical predictions.
   *c. statistical predictions are more reliable than clinical predictions.
   d. neither clinical nor statistical predictions are particularly reliable.

   Page: 31   Topic: Clinical versus Statistical Prediction

57. Which of the following aspects of psychology is the most poorly researched?
   a. diagnosis
   b. treatment
   c. causality
   *d. prevention

   Page: 33   Topic: Could Danielle's Death Have Been Prevented?

58. Primary prevention aims at
   *a. eliminating the cause of a problem and preventing its occurrence.
   b. defining a problem.
   c. identifying and ameliorating the effects of a problem.
   d. treating a problem and rehabilitating individuals with the problem.

   Page: 33   Topic: Primary Prevention

59. The primary prevention of disorders has been impeded by
   a. lack of funds.
   *b. difficulties in defining abnormal behavior.
   c. lack of community concern.
   d. the failure of mental health professionals from different perspectives to cooperate.

   Page: 33   Topic: Primary Prevention

60. Kamal was screened at birth and identified as having PKU. She was immediately placed on a special diet to completely prevent the symptoms of the disorder. This demonstrates
   a. neonatal prevention.
   b. primary prevention.
   *c. secondary prevention.
   d. tertiary prevention.

   Page: 34   Topic: Secondary Prevention

61. The person with the fewest legal rights concerning loss of freedom as a result of a psychological disorder would be
   a. Leandra, a 65-year-old schizophrenic who is homeless.
   b. Myron, a 45-year-old depressed single man who hallucinates.
   c. Nathan, a 25-year-old AIDS patient who is suffering from dementia.
   *d. Olivia, a 15-year-old depressive who is suicidal.

   Page: 35   Topic: Tertiary Prevention

62. Reasons given in the text for prohibiting assisted suicide include all of the following EXCEPT
   *a. that the decision is rightfully God's, not the patient's, the doctor's, or family members'.
   b. fear that this option will be abused.
   c. the possibility that the patient might make such a decision when not thinking clearly.
   d. morality—a doctor's mission is to preserve life, not to end it.

   Page: 36   Topic: Highlight 1.4 Rules for Killing People

63. The debate about physician-assisted suicide has primarily involved all of the following EXCEPT
   a. lawyers.
   *b. psychologists.
   c. doctors.
   d. ethicists.

   Page: 37   Topic: Highlight 1.4 Rules for Killing People

TRUE-FALSE QUESTIONS

64. Although Danielle left no note, all other elements of her death point to the fact that it was a suicide. (F)

    Page: 10   Topic: How Did Danielle Die?

65. Modern clinical psychologists refer to behavior as biopsychosocial. (T)

    Page: 11   Topic: Why Did Danielle Die?

66. With respect to education, a psychologist with a PsyD has been required to complete a more extensive dissertation than a psychologist with a PhD. (F)

    Page: 12   Topic: Highlight 1.1: Who's Who in Mental Health

67. By "biology is destiny," Freud meant that our personalities are strongly determined by whether we are born male or female. (T)

    Page: 11   Topic: Can Depression and Suicidal Behavior Be Inherited?

68. As did the Greeks of Aristotle's time, today's theories attribute depression and suicide to imbalances in body chemistry. (T)

    Page: 15   Topic: Did Danielle's Death Have a Physiological Origin?

69. The term *presentism* refers to how old case studies of psychopathology are presented in modern times so that the average person can understand them. (F)

    Page: 16   Topic: Highlight 1.2: Why We Should Never Judge the Past by the Present

70. The French Royal Commission supported Mesmer's claims that people could be cured of illness with magnetic fluids in tubs filled with iron filings and special water. (F)

    Page: 16   Topic: Mesmerism and the Birth of Modern Abnormal Psychology

71. The interaction of psychological and biological factors is usually sufficient to explain psychopathology. (F)

    Page: 18   Topic: Possible Psychological Contributions to Danielle's Death

72. The wild dancing, head-banging, foaming, and babbling behaviors that were a part of St. Vitus' dance were believed to protect dancers from illness. (T)

    Page: 18   Topic Was Danielle's Death the Result of Social and Cultural Factors?

73. Correlational data about what led a person to suicide can provide strong evidence of causal factors for the suicide. (F)

    Page: 21   Topic: The Cause of Danielle's Death: What Can We Conclude?

74. A person in 19th-century Malaysia who "ran amok" was likely to have been behaving within the guidelines of cultural influences. (T)

    Page: 20   Topic: The Cause of Danielle's Death: What Can We Conclude?

75. Although there is no single agreed-upon definition of abnormality, most mental health professionals do agree on the specific behaviors that constitute abnormality. (F)

    Page: 21   Topic: Was Danielle Mentally Ill?

76. Clinicians overwhelmingly favor categorical descriptions of abnormality because such descriptions facilitate practical application. (T)

    Page: 22   Topic: Danielle's Behavior Was Unusual

11

77. The statistical approach to defining abnormality requires the balancing of costs and benefits. (T)

    Page: 22   Topic: Danielle's Behavior Was Unusual

78. When assessing the results of a suicide lethality test, it is possible to determine with a high degree of certainty which individuals are likely to commit suicide and which individuals are not likely to commit suicide. (F)

    Pages: 22–23   Topic: Critical Thinking About . . . 1.1: How Many Suicides Can We Afford to Prevent?

79. The phrase "acting as *parens patriae*" refers to allowing parents to institutionalize a child if the child's behavior is deemed dangerous to him- or herself or to others. (F)

    Page: 24   Topic: Danielle's Behavior Produced Distress

80. According to utilitarians, behavior is abnormal only when it harms the individual or society. (T)

    Page: 24   Topic: Danielle's Behavior Was Not Functional

81. Functional mental illnesses are those that have a physical basis. (F)

    Page: 27   Topic: General Paresis and Mental Illness

82. In a 1988 British child abuse case, it was possible to differentiate sexually abused children from nonabused children based on abused children's lack of a certain reflex in the muscles of the rectum. (F)

    Page: 31   Topic: Illusory Correlations

83. A serious by-product of information overload for clinicians is overconfidence, which can lead to inaccurate predictions of behavior. (T)

    Page: 31   Topic: Clinical Versus Statistical Prediction

SHORT-ANSWER QUESTIONS

84. Identify the perspective that modern clinical psychologists take toward explaining behavior and the three components of that perspective.

    The biopsychosocial approach states that biological, psychological, and social forces all interact to determine our actions.

    Page: 11   Topic: Why Did Danielle Die?

85. What are the three reasons that historical studies of psychopathology have been more interesting to historians than to clinicians and scientists?

    First, the abstract nature of the studies makes them difficult to understand; second, the studies are unpleasant, abounding in mistreatment, punishment, cruelty, and superstition; and third, obtaining and interpreting original materials is difficult.

    Page: 16   Topic: Highlight 1.2: Why We Should Never Judge the Past by the Present

86. State the problems with imposing the standards of one civilization on another.

    Doing so devalues other times and cultures and denies us the opportunity to learn from them.

    Page: 16   Topic: Highlight 1.2: Why We Should Never Judge the Past by the Present

87. Describe how the six psychological causes most often associated with depression and suicide could be seen in the case of Danielle.

Learned helplessness: she was helpless to stop her father's abuse. Loss of trust: her father's abuse and her mother's complicity could have taught her not to trust others. Guilt and self-blame: she may have felt guilty about her father's suicide and may have felt that in some way she encouraged his sexual abuse of her. Modeling: her father's suicide may have served as a model for her. Loss: her parents' divorce, her father's suicide, and her adoption may all have been linked to her emotional problems. Social isolation: her lack of satisfying social interactions made her more prone to depression and more difficult to treat.

Pages: 17–18   Topic: Possible Psychological Contributions to Danielle's Death

88. Give examples of the three forces that shaped behavior in the Middle Ages that continue to shape behavior today.

Economics: the frequency of psychological disorders increases when unemployment increases. Cultural expectations: today's equating of beauty with being thin may be a reason for the increasing incidence of anorexia nervosa in Western countries. Social stereotypes: people who don't conform to social stereotypes may be isolated and ostracized, which can cause abnormal behavior.

Page: 19   Topic: Was Danielle's Death the Result of Social and Cultural Factors?

89. Discuss the flaws with the statistical approach to abnormality.

First, because they are relative, statistical definitions of abnormality are tied to a particular time and place—what is abnormal in one place may be normal somewhere else; second, this approach can lead to ridiculous conclusions if applied too widely, particularly with desirable extremes such as being too happy or too intelligent.

Page: 22   Topic: Was Danielle's Behavior Unusual?

90. How did politics affect the classification of homosexuality as a psychological disorder?

Homosexuality has, by and large, been prohibited and punished since the rise of Christianity. In this century, the American Psychiatric Association initially disregarded evidence, such as Kinsey's research that homosexuality is too prevalent to be considered an illness and Hooker's findings that homosexuals are as well adjusted as heterosexuals, and classified homosexuality as a disorder. With the emergence of the gay rights movement as a political force in the 1960s, however, the American Psychiatric Association was forced to reconsider its classification of homosexuality as a disorder.

Page: 26   Topic: Critical Thinking About . . . 1.2: Homosexuality and the Politics of Psychiatric Diagnosis

91. Describe the three problems associated with the analogy between medical and psychological illnesses.

Illusory explanations: lacking some independent way to identify the underlying illness, such as a blood test, attributing abnormal behavior to mental illnesses can lead to circular reasoning. Cultural biases: although most physical illnesses are universally recognized, cultural identity is relevant when determining whether a particular behavior, such as suicide, is abnormal. Illness inflation: because there are no objective tests to establish a diagnosis of mental illness, almost anyone who has a problem in life can be classified as mentally ill.

Page: 28   Topic: Differentiating Between Physical and Mental Disorders

92. Explain the four main purposes of a diagnosis.

To provide a convenient way to refer to a syndrome; to provide a focus for research; to suggest an appropriate treatment; to provide prognostic information.

Page: 29   Topic: Why Are Clinical Predictions Often Uncertain?

93. Why are clinical predictions often uncertain?

    Psychiatric diagnoses are full of uncertainties; clinical data are imprecise; test data may be irrelevant or they may have low predictive validity, providing either false-positive or false-negative results.

    Pages: 29–30   Topic: Why Are Clinical Predictions Often Uncertain?

94. How can an assessment device, such as the suicide lethality test, have high predictive validity but low practical value?

    It will miss identifying some individuals who will attempt suicide, but it will also mistakenly classify as suicidal some individuals who will never harm themselves.

    Page: 32   Topic: Critical Thinking About . . . 1.3: Measuring the Practical Value of Psychological Tests

95. What is the potentially serious by-product of information overload for a clinical psychologist, and how is that a problem?

    Information overload produces overconfidence; the more confident clinicians are in the accuracy of their predictions, the more convinced they are that they understand the case, although tests show this does not make them better at predicting outcomes; this suggests clinicians are not always good judges of their own accuracy.

    Page: 31   Topic: Clinical Versus Statistical Prediction

96. How might statistical predictions be more accurate than clinical judgments?

    Statistical formulas are better than unaided clinical judgments in predicting behavior because they are immune to the boredom, fatigue, distraction, and illness that affect human judgments and because they can capture the knowledge of expert clinicians while eliminating their unreliability.

    Page: 31   Topic: Clinical Versus Statistical Prediction

97. How do primary, secondary, and tertiary prevention differ?

    Primary prevention: aims to eliminate the cause of a problem, thereby preventing its occurrence; secondary prevention: aims to identify and ameliorate the problem early in its course; tertiary prevention: deals with treatment and rehabilitation.

    Pages: 33–35   Topic: Could Danielle's Death Have Been Prevented?

98. The various attempts to control costs by determining who will receive treatment and the type of treatment they will receive are known collectively as _____.

    managed care

    Page: 38   Topic: Economics and Prevention

ESSAY QUESTIONS

99. A major section of the chapter discusses whether Danielle was mentally ill. Discuss the five criteria presented, addressing the evidence supporting and criticizing each of these positions.

    Address the issues of behavior being unusual, producing distress, not being functional, and violating social values, and the question of whether her behavior was caused by an illness.

100. Imagine that you hear two classmates arguing about whether there is any point to making a clinical diagnosis and whether clinical predictions are better than statistical predictions. They ask you for your opinion. What would you tell them?

First, discuss the four main purposes of making diagnoses—convenience of reference, focus for research, treatment, and prognostic information—and address the limitations that currently exist in terms of making diagnoses. Then, compare clinical predictions with statistical predictions in terms of how they are made, the problem of overconfidence from having an abundance of information for clinical predictions, and the discussion of how/why statistical predictions may be more accurate than clinical predictions.

101. Consider the issue of false-positives when assessing a potential problem such as suicide. Explain what a false-positive result is and the problems that may result from placing people into discrete categories such as "suicidal" and "not suicidal."

Scores would range along a continuum, for instance, from "not suicidal" to "suicidal," and people who are suicidal would be expected to score higher than those who are not. Depending on where the cutoff point is, some people who are not suicidal may be identified as suicidal—false-positives—and may be hospitalized unnecessarily; conversely, some who actually are suicidal may be missed and may end up committing suicide. This is a cost-benefit analysis in terms of both financial and personal outcomes.

102. As you enter the cafeteria on campus, you hear a loud debate between two of your friends on the politics of psychiatric diagnosis. One friend says that there is no credibility to a diagnosis of something like homosexuality, which is considered abnormal in one time and place and not abnormal in some other time and place. The other friend says that it is the best system we have and that it is sensitive to the cultures in which people live. They ask for your opinion. How would you respond?

This will involve a discussion of changing standards as well as whether psychological disorders disregard scientific evidence—e.g., Kinsey's and Hooker's respective research. A good answer will also look at the political aspects of diagnoses; social acceptance of certain behaviors; and, as in the case of homosexuality, whether those exhibiting certain behaviors are—or are not—well adjusted. Finally, in terms of assessing whether any particular set of behaviors is abnormal, it is important to look at the entire population exhibiting those behaviors, not just those who are seeking help for their emotional problems, to determine whether people with those behaviors are having problems of adjustment.

103. Considering all that you have read about the case of Danielle Woods, discuss how her death might have been prevented.

This answer requires a review of primary, secondary, and tertiary prevention strategies and how they would apply to Danielle's experience.

CHAPTER 2
PARADIGMS AND PERSPECTIVES, MODELS AND METHODS

MULTIPLE-CHOICE QUESTIONS

1. Theoretical frameworks determine all of the following EXCEPT
   *a. the way we test a hypothesis about behavior.
   b. how we approach the task of understanding others.
   c. the viewpoints that we adopt.
   d. the data that we perceive.

   Page: 42   Topic: Introduction

2. A _____ is the conceptual framework within which a scientist works.
   a. theory
   *b. paradigm
   c. model
   d. hypothesis

   Page: 42   Topic: Introduction

3. The paradigm that emphasizes how early experience and unconscious conflicts can cause abnormal behavior
   is the _____ paradigm.
   a. behavioral
   b. biological
   *c. psychoanalytic
   d. cognitive

   Page: 42   Topic: Introduction

4. Dr. Amherst works with her clients by focusing on their pathological thinking to help alleviate their
   psychological problems. Which approach does Dr. Amherst use?
   a. biological
   b. psychoanalytic
   c. behavioral
   *d. cognitive

   Page: 42   Topic: Introduction

5. The metaparadigm used in abnormal psychology
   *a. provides coherence in what might otherwise appear to be a chaotic field.
   b. demonstrates the inherent conflict among the various paradigms.
   c. attempts to provide a single, clear explanation of behavior.
   d. demonstrates the competition among the various paradigms.

   Page: 43   Topic: Abnormal Psychology's Metaparadigm

6. The first step in investigating the hypothesis that heredity plays a role in behavior disorders is to
   a. interview and do psychological assessments of people with the particular disorder.
   *b. perform a pedigree study in which the family trees of probands are searched for relatives with similar
   disorders.
   c. determine which theoretical paradigm would be most appropriate.
   d. determine the specific type of data analysis that will be used once the data are collected.

   Page: 45   Topic: Pedigree Studies

7. Individuals with a particular disorder that is under investigation are referred to as
   a. participants.
   b. subjects.
   *c. probands.
   d. cases.

   Page: 45   Topic: Pedigree Studies

8. In the case discussed in the text, Danielle behaved
   a. more like her adoptive father than her natural father, thus suggesting the greater influence of environment than genetics.
   *b. more like her natural father than her adoptive father, thus suggesting the greater influence of genetics than environment.
   c. in many ways like her adoptive father, but in other ways like her natural father, thus suggesting the mutual strength of both environment and genetics.
   d. more like her adoptive mother than like either of her natural parents, thus suggesting the greater influence of environment than genetics.

   Page: 47   Topic: Twin Studies

9. The most powerful adoption studies involve
   a. dizygotic twins reared together.
   b. monozygotic twins reared together.
   c. dizygotic twins reared apart.
   *d. monozygotic twins reared apart.

   Page: 47   Topic: Twin Studies

10. Amanda, who has recently attempted suicide, is now in therapy. Not only has her therapist interviewed her, but the clinician has also interviewed her relatives and examined her previous clinical records. The therapist will be faced with problems in getting an unbiased view of Amanda for all of the following reasons EXCEPT:
    *a. the previous therapist is likely to refuse to release information, despite Amanda's consent.
    b. Amanda and her relatives are likely to engage in selective forgetting.
    c. Amanda and her relatives are likely to lie outright to avoid blame and guilt.
    d. the clinical data may have been recorded by a therapist with a biased viewpoint.

    Page: 48   Topic: Prospective Studies

11. All of the following are problems with prospective studies EXCEPT:
    a. they are expensive and take a long time.
    *b. it is difficult to identify potential participants.
    c. many children are incorrectly included in high-risk groups.
    d. many children who are high risk will be lost to the study because their families move.

    Page: 48   Topic: Prospective Studies

12. Once biochemistry becomes highly sophisticated in terms of molecular genetics, psychologists will
    a. be able to isolate the gene that is most responsible for depression.
    b. use biochemical techniques to predict who will develop depression.
    *c. still need to understand the role of the environment in the development of depression.
    d. come to rely on genetic maps to predict who will develop depression.

    Page: 49   Topic: Prospective Studies

13. The text notes that a great irony of eugenics is that
    a. although we faulted Nazi Germany for pursuing the "perfect race," eugenics is now being used in the United States to create "perfect" babies.
    b. the idea originated with Charles Darwin, with his notion of survival of the fittest.
    c. based on the ideas inherent in eugenics, millions of people have died in the pursuit of a "perfect race."
    *d. by assuming that genetically transmitted traits are immutable, eugenicists ignore the fact that phenotypes are affected by both biological and environmental factors.

    Pages: 50–51   Topic: Highlight 2.1: Do Only the Strong Deserve to Survive?

14. With respect to heritability, all of the following hypotheses have found at least limited support EXCEPT:
    *a. there are molecular differences between suicidal and nonsuicidal people.
    b. suicide occurs more commonly in the families of suicidal people.
    c. suicide occurs more frequently in close relatives of those who commit suicide than in their distant relatives.
    d. adopted children resemble their natural parents more than their adoptive parents.

    Page: 49   Topic: Prospective Studies

15. Calling the biological paradigm a medical model confuses the distal biological causes of behavior with all of the following EXCEPT
    a. economic issues.
    *b. medical evaluations.
    c. social issues.
    d. legal judgments.

    Page: 51   Topic: Biological Paradigm Question 2: Is Abnormal Behavior a Disease?

16. The most prevalent scientific method is
    a. correlational studies.
    b. controlled experiments.
    *c. naturalistic observation.
    d. participant observation.

    Page: 52   Topic: Naturalistic Observation

17. All of the following are true about case studies EXCEPT:
    a. they are psychology's most commonly used type of naturalistic observation.
    b. they have given rise to important research programs.
    c. they are difficult to generalize.
    *d. they provide unbiased information.

    Page: 52   Topic: Naturalistic Observation

18. Dr. Adelson has found a correlation between the eating of chocolate and positive mood. Based on this finding, he might safely conclude that
    *a. a third variable might cause people to eat chocolate and to be in a positive mood.
    b. eating chocolate causes people to be in a positive mood.
    c. being in a positive mood may cause people to eat chocolate.
    d. the relationship is cyclical—eating chocolate puts people in a positive mood, and people in a positive mood then eat more chocolate.

    Page: 52   Topic: Correlational Studies

19. When investigating the effects of reserpine on levels of norepinephrine (which is related to depression), a research team administered reserpine to one group of nondepressed participants in a study, while another group was given a placebo. The independent variable in that study was the
   a. placebo.
   *b. reserpine.
   c. norepinephrine.
   d. depression.

   Page: 52   Topic: Controlled Studies

20. Dr. Emerson is studying the effects of reserpine on levels of norepinephrine. She is concerned that if a member of her research team knows which participants are receiving the reserpine, the team member might expect those participants to become depressed and would thus show more concern for those participants than for participants receiving the placebo. Because of this possibility, Dr. Emerson would not be able to tell if any differences she saw in her groups were due to the reserpine or to their being treated differently. To avoid this, Dr. Emerson will
   a. fully train all members of her research team on how to work with the participants.
   b. debrief her participants after the study to see if this was a problem.
   *c. use a double-blind study to avoid the problem.
   d. have the reserpine administered by a machine.

   Page: 53   Topic: Controlled Studies

21. In order that participants in a study are able to provide voluntary, informed consent,
   a. participants must know precisely what the researcher is studying.
   b. the researcher must have custodial persons (e.g., parents, teachers) tell participants what is involved in the research.
   c. a standard format must be developed to inform all participants about the potential risks and benefits of the study.
   *d. participants must be informed of the potential risks and benefits of the study, and they must have the capacity to consent.

   Page: 53   Topic: Ethical Challenges

22. Ethical considerations in research require all of the following EXCEPT:
   *a. no deception of participants about research goals.
   b. voluntary, informed consent.
   c. potential benefits that outweigh potential risks.
   d. participant anonymity.

   Page: 53   Topic: Ethical Challenges

23. Dr. Parks is researching the relationship between child abuse and later suicide. Because it would be highly unethical for her to subject children to abuse intentionally for the purposes of her study, she would probably most likely try to seek support for her theory by
   a. conducting an analogue experiment.
   *b. accumulating correlational evidence.
   c. interviewing adults who survived suicide attempts.
   d. identifying abusive families and observing the children as they develop.

   Page: 55   Topic: Accumulating Evidence

24. The relationship between reserpine and depression has been supported by which of the following findings?
    a. Neurotransmitters other than norepinephrine have been implicated as possible causes of depression.
    b. Monamine oxidase inhibitors (MAOs) decrease the amount of norepinephrine in certain neurons.
    *c. Tricyclic antidepressant drugs increase the amount of norepinephrine in certain neurons.
    d. Hypertensive patients receiving reserpine have experienced increased levels of norepinephrine.

    Page: 55   Topic: Accumulating Evidence

25. When Freud first began working with patients who suffered from hysteria, he used
    a. hypnosis.
    b. talk therapy.
    c. analysis of dreams and resistance.
    *d. rest, baths, and electric currents.

    Page: 55   Topic: Sigmund Freud: Hysteria, Hypnosis, and the Unconscious

26. When working with Anna O., Breuer realized the importance of _____ for helping patients work through their traumatic experiences.
    *a. catharsis
    b. hypnosis
    c. repression
    d. confrontation

    Page: 56   Topic: Sigmund Freud: Hysteria, Hypnosis, and the Unconscious

27. Freud and Breuer determined that some childhood traumas are too disturbing to be admitted into consciousness, so they are kept unconscious through a process called
    a. suppression.
    *b. repression.
    c. denial.
    d. displacement.

    Page: 56   Topic: Sigmund Freud: Hysteria, Hypnosis, and the Unconscious

28. When in her psychology class, Leilani focuses on her professor's lecture. If her professor were to stop and ask his students to state their name and birthdates, they would easily be able to do so. That is because this information is stored at the _____ level of awareness.
    a. conscious
    b. unconscious
    *c. preconscious
    d. subconscious

    Page: 56   Topic: Psychoanalytic Paradigm Question 1: What Is the Personality . . .

29. When unconscious material reaches consciousness, the material usually is
    a. viewed as a great insight.
    b. acknowledged as important to healing.
    c. experienced with relief.
    *d. experienced as foreign.

    Page: 57   Topic: Psychoanalytic Paradigm Question 1: What Is the Personality . . .

30. The id satisfies its wish-fulfilling fantasies through _____ process thinking.
    *a. primary-
    b. secondary-
    c. pleasure-
    d. anticipatory-

    Page: 57   Topic: Psychoanalytic Paradigm Question 1: What Is the Personality . . .

31. One of the superego's responsibilities is to
    a. strike a compromise between the id, the ego, and the real world.
    *b. set a moral code to guide the individual's behavior.
    c. quickly achieve gratification of the individual's biological needs.
    d. satisfy needs without violating the demands of civilized society.

    Page: 57   Topic: Psychoanalytic Paradigm Question 1: What Is the Personality . . .

32. Sally told Harry that his *libido* was overactive. If she used the term correctly, she would be referring to the psychological "energy" Harry derived from his
    a. death instinct.
    b. aggressive tendencies.
    *c. life instincts.
    d. dynamic processes.

    Page: 57   Topic: Psychoanalytic Paradigm Question 1: What Is the Personality . . .

33. Floyd was frustrated in his attempts to achieve pleasure from sucking and eating during his first few months of life, resulting in fixation during this stage. According to the Freudian theory of psychosexual development, we would expect that
    a. when Floyd has children, he will be likely to see that this does not happen to them.
    b. as an adult, Floyd is likely to engage in a lifelong rebellion against society.
    c. Floyd is likely never to be able to adopt a mature adult sexual role.
    *d. Floyd is likely to engage in such activities as smoking and eating "junk" food as an adult.

    Page: 58   Topic: The Psychosexual Stages

34. The superego develops during the _____ stage.
    *a. phallic
    b. genital
    c. oral
    d. anal

    Page: 58   Topic: The Psychosexual Stages

35. Freud suggested all of the following concerning the connection between anxiety and repression EXCEPT:
    a. unconscious repressed material creates anxiety.
    *b. allowing repressed material into conscious awareness reduces anxiety.
    c. repression is a way of protecting the ego.
    d. repression is rarely successful at protecting the ego.

    Page: 58   Topic: Anxiety and Defense

36. Freud based his theory of psychosexual development on his work with primarily
    a. working-class Viennese men.
    b. young Viennese children and adolescents.
    *c. middle-class Viennese women.
    d. the patients he studied in France who suffered from hysteria.

    Page: 58   Topic: Anxiety and Defense

37. Margaret has finally tired of her husband's periodic binges. Every 3 months, before he gets paid, Dan starts an argument with her, which he believes justifies his taking his paycheck and spending it on drinks for himself and his "friends" at the local bar. After bailing Dan out of jail for the fourth time after one of these binges, Margaret finally gets him to a meeting of Alcoholics Anonymous. Dan stands up and says, "Hi. My name is Dan. I am *not* an alcoholic." Which defense mechanism is Dan exhibiting?
   a. reaction formation
   b. rationalization
   c. sublimation
   *d. denial

   Page: 59   Topic: Anxiety and Defense

38. The defense mechanism that Freud believed had the least amount of reality distortion and the greatest amount of social value is
   *a. sublimation.
   b. reaction formation.
   c. repression.
   d. rationalization.

   Page: 59   Topic: Anxiety and Defense

39. The technique Freud developed that requires patients to produce whatever comes into their minds, no matter how irrelevant or nonsensical, is referred to as
   a. hypnotic trance.
   *b. free association.
   c. talk therapy.
   d. deep concentration.

   Page: 60   Topic: Psychoanalytic Paradigm Question 2: How Should Psychological Disorders Be Treated?

40. Freud used all of the following techniques in his therapy EXCEPT
   a. dream interpretation.
   b. interpretation of transference.
   *c. mesmerism.
   d. free association.

   Page: 60   Topic: Psychoanalytic Paradigm Question 2: How Should Psychological Disorders Be Treated?

41. Dr. Santos is working with 18-year-old Anthony, who has recently graduated from high school and is now trying to make important life choices about his career, his social commitments, and the type of person he should become. This would most closely reflect whose perspective?
   *a. Erikson's identity crisis
   b. Freud's resolution of the Oedipal conflict
   c. Adler's notion of striving for superiority
   d. Jung's emphasis on the need for self-actualization

   Page: 62   Topic: Modifications to Psychoanalysis by Neo- and Post-Freudians

42. In Freud's famous case of the Rat Man, the patient's obsessive-compulsive symptoms were ultimately attributed by Freud to the patient's
   a. uncomfortable relationship with his girlfriend.
   *b. ambivalent relationship with his father.
   c. desire to be released from the army.
   d. fear of a sadistic senior officer in the army.

   Page: 63   Topic: The Evolution of a Psychoanalytic Hypothesis

43. Most psychologists today tend to agree with Freud on all of the following EXCEPT
    a. the importance of childhood experiences.
    b. the existence of unconscious motivation.
    *c. the validity of internal consistency as a measure of effective outcome.
    d. the belief that behavior disorders result from anxiety and conflicts.

    Page: 64   Topics: The Evolution of a Psychoanalytic Hypothesis; Psychoanalytic Paradigm: Current Status

44. Wilhelm was participating in an experiment that required him to describe his own subjective experiences of a purple hat (including all of his physical sensations and internal thoughts). This would be most likely associated with which school of psychology?
    a. psychoanalytic
    b. humanistic
    c. functionalist
    *d. structuralist

    Page: 65   Topic: Behavioral Paradigm Question 1: What Are the Basic Elements of Behavior?

45. In developing the new view of behaviorism, John B. Watson believed that
    *a. all behavior is learned through experience.
    b. human behavior is learned through experience, but animal behavior is in large part instinctive.
    c. much of human and animal behavior is instinctive, but all we can really study is observable behavior.
    d. behavior that is reinforced will be repeated.

    Page: 66   Topic: Behavioral Paradigm Question 1: What Are the Basic Elements of Behavior?

46. In Pavlov's classical conditioning paradigm, the CS produces
    a. a response opposite to the response produced by the UCS.
    *b. a response similar to the response produced by the UCS.
    c. fear.
    d. salivation.

    Page: 66   Topic: The Conditioned Reflex

47. The text noted all of the following about Watson and Rayner's Little Albert experiment EXCEPT:
    a. it was designed as an alternative to Freud's explanation of the development of phobias.
    b. it contained methodological errors.
    *c. Little Albert's fear generalized from fear of the rat to all things white and furry.
    d. Watson and Rayner exaggerated Little Albert's "fear" of other furry objects.

    Page: 68   Topic: Behavioral Paradigm Question 2: Can Psychological Symptoms Be Learned?

48. Watson believed that cognitive processes _____, whereas Skinner believed that they _____.
    a. are tangentially important; are irrelevant.
    b. are irrelevant; are tangentially important.
    c. should be considered as stimuli; should be considered as responses.
    *d. should be ignored; do not exist.

    Page: 69   Topic: Operant Conditioning

49. Thorndike's "law of effect" states that behavior that
    *a. leads to favorable outcomes will be repeated.
    b. leads to negative outcomes will be abandoned.
    c. requires more than one or two cognitive steps cannot be learned by lower animals.
    d. is not continually reinforced will be abandoned.

    Page: 69   Topic: Operant Conditioning

50. All of the following may be explained by operant conditioning EXCEPT
    a. pigeons learning to play Ping-Pong.
    *b. students learning to type.
    c. pathological gambling.
    d. compulsive behavior.

    Page: 70   Topic: Operant Conditioning

51. The text presented a newspaper article about the suicide attempt by Millicent Pommeroy, a friend of Danielle Wood. This was explained in terms of
    a. classical conditioning.
    b. operant conditioning.
    *c. modeling.
    d. mediated learning.

    Pages: 70–71   Topic: Modeling

52. Avoidance learning is known as the two-process theory because it is based on both
    a. modeling and classical conditioning.
    b. modeling and operant conditioning.
    c. operant conditioning and mediated learning.
    *d. classical conditioning and operant conditioning.

    Page: 71   Topic: Mediated Learning

53. Lexter, a lineman for the telephone company, had suddenly developed acrophobia. This fear of heights was keeping him from performing those duties that required him to climb phone poles to work on phone lines. To get over this phobia, Lexter forced himself to climb to the top of a phone pole and remain there until his anxiety symptoms stopped. This technique is known as
    *a. flooding.
    b. systematic desensitization.
    c. behavior modification.
    d. counterconditioning.

    Page: 72   Topic: Behavioral Paradigm Question 3: Can Psychological Disorders Be Unlearned?

54. What is a primary difference between the methodology used to support Seligman's theory of learned helplessness and Freud's psychoanalytic theory?
    a. Freud based his theory on the case studies of his adult patients, whereas Seligman based his theory on his work with children.
    *b. Freud's theory was essentially immune to refutation, whereas Seligman looked for corroborating evidence from a variety of sources.
    c. Freud based his theory solely on his work with humans, whereas Seligman based his theory solely on his work with animals.
    d. Freud's conclusions were based on empirical research, whereas Seligman's conclusions were based on scientific research.

    Page: 75   Topic: Comparison with Psychoanalysis

55. The modern cognitive psychologists have turned what was formerly a mentalistic pseudoscience into an objective, scientific enterprise by
    a. making extensive clinical observations.
    b. using CT scans and other physiological measures.
    *c. inferring mental concepts from objective behavior.
    d. meticulously recording individual perceptions.

    Page: 76   Topic: Cognitive Paradigm Question 1: Can Cognition Be Studied Scientifically?

56. Inferences that we make about the causes of events, our own behavior, and the behavior of others are referred to as
    a. appraisals.
    b. expectancies.
    c. beliefs.
    *d. attributions.

    Page: 76   Topic: Cognitive Paradigm Question 2: How Do We Construe Our World?

57. Xavier explained to his parents, "I didn't make the basketball team because I'm not good enough at any sport, and I never will be." This would demonstrate which constellation of attributions?
    *a. internal, permanent, and global
    b. internal, permanent, and specific
    c. internal, temporary, and global
    d. external, permanent, and global

    Page: 77   Topic: Cognitive Paradigm Question 2: How Do We Construe Our World?

58. How does Ellis say that beliefs differ from appraisals and attributions?
    a. They are specific to particular social situations.
    *b. They represent a person's characteristic mode of thinking.
    c. They are typically irrational.
    d. They are more precise.

    Page: 78   Topic: Beliefs

59. At the beginning of fifth grade, Miss Hecker is told that certain children in her class are exceptionally bright. Although these children were selected at random, based on the research in this area, what would we expect to see by the end of the school year?
    a. Miss Hecker will figure out that there are no major differences between these children and the other children in the class.
    b. Miss Hecker will decide that these children need less attention and thus will focus on other children who (she believes) need her help more.
    *c. Miss Hecker will treat these children in such a way that they will, in fact, excel in their studies.
    d. Miss Hecker will figure out which children are really the brightest and will focus her attention on those children, ensuring their success.

    Page: 80   Topic: Generalize and Seek Corroborating Evidence

60. Dr. Karl believes human beings are independent agents, free to make choices and to control their own destinies. We may safely assume that Dr. Karl holds a _____ perspective.
    a. behavioristic
    b. psychoanalytic
    c. cognitive
    *d. humanistic

    Page: 81   Topic: Humanistic Paradigm

61. The humanistic paradigm differs from the existential paradigm in that the humanistic paradigm
    *a. views the world optimistically.
    b. finds meaning in life.
    c. enhances human dignity.
    d. helps people make choices about their behavior.

    Page: 81   Topic: Humanistic Paradigm

62. From a humanistic perspective, Danielle's psychological problems may have arisen, at least in part, from
    a. being overprotected by her adoptive mother.
    *b. trying to ensure that others would love her.
    c. being sexually molested as a child.
    d. trying too hard to succeed.

    Page: 82   Topic: Humanistic Paradigm Question 2: How Can We Help People to Self-Actualize?

63. Dr. Abraham, a humanistic therapist, would most likely treat
    a. Arnold, who has been hospitalized twice for schizophrenia.
    b. Bruce, who has a severe phobia of rodents and insects.
    *c. Carl, who feels he is not achieving his true potential.
    d. Daniel, who has suffered from bipolar disorder for the past year.

    Page: 82   Topic: Humanistic Paradigm Question 3: How Can We Help People to Self-Actualize?

64. Mr. and Mrs. Jones have told their therapist that they argue with each other between 2 and 3 hours a day. Their therapist has told them they need to increase their daily arguments to 5 hours. The therapist is using which therapeutic technique?
    a. unconditional positive regard
    b. accurate empathy
    c. conflict analysis
    *d. paradoxical intention

    Page: 83   Topic: Humanistic Paradigm Question 3: How Can We Help People to Self-Actualize?

65. The humanistic paradigm has been criticized for all of the following EXCEPT:
    *a. it is not effective in helping people with their emotional problems.
    b. it is vague, unscientific, and overly simplistic.
    c. humanistic ideas are not much different from behavioral and cognitive ideas.
    d. all therapeutic paradigms attempt to help people who suffer, so they are all humanistic approaches.

    Pages: 83–84   Topic: Humanistic Paradigm: Current Status

66. Dr. Wu has noticed that her objective findings about several patients indicate they are all more or less equally healthy. The patients' subjective reports of their health differ greatly, however, depending on their ethnic background. Because Dr. Wu considers these subjective differences to be important in treating her patients, she is using a _____ paradigm.
    a. humanistic
    *b. sociocultural
    c. biomedical
    d. cognitive

    Page: 85   Topic: Sociocultural Paradigm

67. The high incidence of anorexia nervosa among teenage women in Western society demonstrates the strong influence of
    a. cultural interpretations.
    b. acculturation stress.
    *c. cultural stereotypes.
    d. sex role stereotypes.

    Page: 85   Topic: Cultural Stereotypes

68. What event appeared to shift the persecution for witchcraft from both men and women almost entirely to women?
    a. the papal bull of Pope Innocent VIII
    b. the Crusades
    c. publication of the Gutenberg Bible
    *d. publication of the *Malleus Maleficarum*

    Page: 88   Topic: Highlight 2.3: Witches and Victimization

69. According to the sociocultural paradigm, who is most likely to experience a deterioration of her psychological health?
    *a. Zena, a single mother. She moved to New York with her son to take a job she loved but got laid off from her job 18 months ago.
    b. Yetta, a teenager. She lives with her parents and was let go from her job at a fast-food restaurant last month.
    c. Xanath, a 65-year-old grandmother. She retired from her job 6 months ago and has been traveling with her husband ever since.
    d. Wanda, a 30-year-old single woman. She hated her job since she started there, and since she was laid off three months ago, she has been volunteering at the Red Cross.

    Pages: 89–90   Topic: The Evolution of a Sociocultural Hypothesis

TRUE-FALSE QUESTIONS

70. All of the current paradigms of abnormal psychology take for granted that the immediate causes of behavior are biological. (T)

    Page: 43   Topic: Abnormal Psychology's Metaparadigm

71. All scientists working in the field of abnormal psychology begin by observing behavior. (T)

    Page: 45   Topic: Biological Paradigm

72. By examining identical twins reared together, it is possible to determine the extent to which heredity contributes to a particular behavior disorder. (F)

    Page: 47   Topic: Twin Studies

73. The belief that behavior disorders are biological in origin and best left to doctors to treat dominates modern medicine because researchers have found biological causes for the majority of behavior disorders. (F)

    Page: 49   Topic: Biological Paradigm Question 2: Is Abnormal Behavior a Disease?

74. The use of medical terminology for behavior disorders does not necessarily reflect an illness model. (T)

    Page: 49   Topic: Biological Paradigm Question 2: Is Abnormal Behavior a Disease?

75. In general, there has been a trend in the psychodynamic approach to focus less on biological instincts and more on the social determinants of personality development. (T)

    Page: 61   Topic: Modifications to Psychoanalysis by Neo- and Post-Freudians

76. Behaviorism is a theory directed specifically at observable behaviors. (F)

    Page: 65   Topic: Behavioral Paradigm

77. Extinction is the same thing as forgetting. (F)

    Page: 70   Topic: Operant Conditioning

78. According to Skinner, punishment results in only a temporary inhibition of behavior. (T)

Page: 70   Topic: Operant Conditioning

79. The success of various forms of behavioral treatment demonstrates that behavioral explanations for the etiology of various pathological conditions are likely to be correct. (F)

Page: 72   Topic: Behavioral Paradigm Question 3: Can Psychological Disorders Be Unlearned?

80. Because longitudinal studies are expensive, retrospective studies provide an effective substitute. (F)

Page: 74   Topic: Critical Thinking About . . . 2.1: Just Because You Are Dead . . .

81. Whereas behaviorists see enuresis (bed-wetting) as a learning problem, Freudian psychologists see it as a symptom of an underlying sexual conflict. (T)

Page: 73   Topic: Highlight 2.2: Is Bed-Wetting a Symptom or an Illness?

82. The methodology of modern cognitive psychology is more similar to the methodology of classical geneticists than to that of the structuralists. (T)

Page: 76   Topic: Cognitive Paradigm Question 1: Can Cognition Be Studied Scientifically?

83. In Lazarus's study of participants watching Australian Aboriginal boys being circumcised, participants who were told the boys were not distressed by the initiation rite were more stressed than participants who were told the boys were suffering. (F)

Page: 78   Topic: Appraisals

84. Ellis's "beliefs" are similar to "attributions" in that when faulty, both may be responsible for psychological disorders. (T)

Page: 78   Topic: Beliefs

85. According to Bandura, expectancies develop from vicarious learning. (T)

Page: 79   Topic: The Evolution of a Cognitive Hypothesis

86. The cognitive paradigm represents a radical departure from behaviorism. (F)

Page: 80   Topic: Cognitive Paradigm: Current Status

87. The humanistic paradigm is one of the most extensively researched of the various psychotherapeutic paradigms. (F)

Page: 82   Topic: Humanistic Paradigm Question 3: How Can We Help People to Self-Actualize?

88. Acculturation always involves some degree of stress. (F)

Page: 87   Topic: Acculturation Stress

89. The goal of the sociocultural paradigm is to describe and understand how culture interacts with universal biological and psychological traits. (T)

Page: 91   Topic: Sociocultural Paradigm: Current Status

SHORT-ANSWER QUESTIONS

90. Describe the two causes of behavior that explain how paradigms other than the biological paradigm can be used to explain behavior.

    Proximal (immediate) causes of behavior can always be found in the activity of the central nervous system and its associated organs (e.g., muscles, glands) at any point in time. The state of the central nervous system is the result of distal (distant) factors that include heredity, early life experiences, as well as other social and psychological influences.

    Page: 43   Topic: Abnormal Psychology's Metaparadigm

91. Briefly describe the six paradigms of abnormal psychology and how they produce behavior.

    The proximal cause of behavior is activity in the central nervous system and its effectors. Distal factors affect the central nervous system, leading, in turn, to the proximal factors. Biological paradigm: genetics, illness, disease, drug effects, toxicity. Psychoanalytic paradigm: early experience, unconscious conflict. Behavioral paradigm: learned habits. Cognitive paradigm: attitudes and attributions. Humanistic paradigm: values, faulty self-concept. Sociocultural paradigm: cultural rules.

    Pages: 43–44   Topic: Abnormal Psychology's Metaparadigm

92. Explain why it is so difficult to determine the extent to which heredity contributes to a particular behavior disorder, even when studying monozygotic twins reared apart.

    Even separated twins may grow up in similar environments because social service agencies try to place children in homes similar to their natural ones and because many children are adopted by relatives. Finding monozygotic twins reared in dissimilar environments from early in life is rare. Further, it is not known which aspects of the environment are important causes of specific mental disorders such as depression.

    Page: 47   Topic: Twin Studies

93. What are the two reasons stated in the text for characterizing the biological paradigm as a medical model of abnormal behavior?

    First, those who work in the biological paradigm tend to use medical terms (e.g., syndrome, diagnosis). Second, it is often assumed that behavior disorders that have their roots in biology are, by definition, illnesses that should be managed by health care professionals.

    Page: 49   Topic: Biological Paradigm Question 2: Is Abnormal Behavior a Disease?

94. If researchers were to find that homosexuality is a biological rather than a social phenomenon, would this discovery mean that the American Psychiatric Association was wrong and that homosexuality is a disease after all?

    No. If homosexuality has a neurophysiological cause, so would heterosexuality. To be logically consistent, heterosexuality would also have to be called an illness because it is caused biologically.

    Pages: 49–50   Topic: Biological Paradigm Question 2: Is Abnormal Behavior a Disease?

95. What two ideas form the cornerstone of Freud's theory of psychosexual stages of development?

    People are born savages and must be socialized to behave morally; and sexual identity is not innate, but develops out of early family experience.

    Page: 58   Topic: Personality Development

96. How did the theories of Jung, Erikson, and Adler differ from Freud's theory?

Unlike Freud, who emphasized sex drives and the influence of early childhood experiences, Jung stressed people's ability to set and meet goals and the influence of the collective unconscious (a genetic data bank we inherit from our ancestors); Adler stressed the human need to "strive for superiority" in some aspect of life; and Erikson proposed a lifespan approach and stressed the social environment. All three also differed from Freud in their more optimistic view of human beings.

Page: 61   Topic: Modifications to Psychoanalysis by Neo- and Post-Freudians

97. Explain Watson's excitement about Pavlov's research.

It was a way for Watson to convince his fellow psychologists that behaviorism was a viable paradigm for psychology in that conditioning not only provided a research program and a research method, but also a way to demonstrate behaviorism's superiority to psychoanalysis.

Page: 69   Topic: The Conditioned Reflex

98. Describe Skinner's view of the difference between negative reinforcement and punishment.

Negative reinforcement refers to the removal of a noxious stimulus on the emission of an operant, and leads to learning. Punishment refers to following a behavior with a noxious stimulus, and results in a temporary inhibition of behavior. As soon as the punishment is removed, the behavior returns.

Page: 69   Topic: Operant Conditioning

99. Describe Wolpe's treatment of systematic desensitization and explain the two Pavlovian conditioning processes at work in that treatment.

Wolpe's systematic desensitization requires the phobic person to imagine a series of gradually more frightening scenes (the anxiety hierarchy) while at the same time trying to relax as deeply as possible. The two Pavlovian conditioning processes are extinction, which occurs because of the repeated presentation of feared situations (the CS) without any unpleasant consequences (i.e., without a UCS), and new conditioning, with relaxation replacing fear as the response to feared scenes.

Page: 72   Topic: Behavioral Paradigm Question 3: Can Psychological Disorders Be Unlearned?

100. What is one way in which Seligman's theory of learned helplessness has been revised to account for specific characteristics of depressed people, such as self-blame and whether people do or do not get better over time?

A distinction was made between universal helplessness (events beyond an individual's control) and personal helplessness (events within a person's control). Both can cause depression, but only the second produces self-blame and becomes chronic; depression from universal helplessness dissipates quickly.

Page: 74   Topic: Revisions Based on More Precise Observations

101. Describe Ellis's rational-emotive therapy.

RET is designed to expose and challenge an individual's irrational beliefs. Using a combination of logical argument, modeling, and a variety of other techniques, Ellis attempts to get people to abandon the unreasonable "shoulds" and "musts" that keep them from leading fulfilling lives.

Page: 79   Topic: Beliefs

102. Explain the two general types of expectancies identified by Bandura.

An outcome expectancy is a person's belief that a behavior will lead to a particular outcome; efficacy expectancies are beliefs about one's personal ability to execute a behavior. If people have low efficacy expectations, they may limit their lives and avoid situations where they expect to fail; those with high efficacy expectations will try and keep on trying, and may even try harder when faced with a tough challenge.

Page: 79   Topic: The Evolution of a Cognitive Hypothesis

103. Describe the three ways stated in the text that the behavioral and cognitive paradigms are similar.

    First, like behaviorists, cognitive psychologists are reductionists who break complex behaviors down into simpler constituents; second, they stress the importance of objective measures of behavior and of testing theories empirically; third, if the stimulus-response relationship is construed as the relationship between antecedent conditions and behavior, then those working in the cognitive paradigm have the same goals as the behaviorists—both want to describe, predict, and control the antecedent conditions that determine human behavior.

    Page: 80   Topic: Cognitive Paradigm: Current Status

104. With respect to their focus on the individual, what is the primary way in which behaviorists and humanists differ?

    Behaviorists focus on the similarities among people; humanists focus on the self as psychology's main subject matter, thus emphasizing the uniqueness of each individual.

    Pages: 81–82   Topic: Humanistic Paradigm Question 1: What Is the Proper Subject of Psychology?

ESSAY QUESTIONS

105. As you come into the cafeteria at the student union, several of your classmates ask you to join them. They are arguing about which psychological paradigm best explains what happened to Danielle, the student described in the book who apparently committed suicide. They ask you what you think of each of the paradigms, and how each explains what happened to Danielle. How would you respond?

    This requires discussion of each of the paradigms (biological, psychoanalytic, behavioral, cognitive, humanistic, and sociocultural) and how each would apply to the case of Danielle.

106. Imagine that you have a young, school-aged cousin who is experiencing problems with enuresis. The boy's mother wants to punish him for wetting the bed, but the father thinks the child just needs to "grow out of it." They turn to you for advice. Describe to them the difference between enuresis as an illness to be cured or as a symptom of some deeper issues. What would you advise them to do?

    This entails a comparison of how the behavioral and psychoanalytic perspectives would each approach this problem, including how to deal with it effectively.

107. You have just taken a job working in an after-school day care center. You have noticed, among this ethnically diverse group of children, three youngsters who seem to be especially withdrawn. You learn that they are siblings who have recently come to the United States with their parents, who were forced to leave their native country. What paradigm would best help you understand and work with these children?

    A discussion of the sociocultural paradigm, particularly focusing on acculturation stress, is called for.

108. While volunteering at a local hospital, you have begun to notice something interesting. Those patients who appear to get most easily agitated, and who seem to scream at the nurses and orderlies, seem to have high blood pressure. You come to believe that screaming and being easily agitated actually cause high blood pressure. Discuss the defect in this conclusion.

    A discussion of how correlation does not infer causation and how some third variable may be causing both variables is appropriate.

109. One of your classmates has just committed suicide. As you are discussing this with other members of your class, someone says, "You know, someone who is so weak they can't take the pressure shouldn't be encouraged to live anyway. Spencer and Darwin were right—it really should be survival of the fittest. We should let the poor and the lunatics disappear, and then we'll get rid of all poverty and illness and all those mentally defective people who are running around shooting themselves and others." How would you respond?

This requires a look at the work of Darwin and Spencer (noting that it was Spencer, not Darwin, who coined the phrase "survival of the fittest"), as well as a look at Nazi Germany, and then a discussion of how genotype and phenotype are confused and played out.

CHAPTER 3
PSYCHOLOGICAL ASSESSMENT, CLASSIFICATION, AND CLINICAL DECISION MAKING

MULTIPLE-CHOICE QUESTIONS

1. Psychological assessments include all of the following EXCEPT
   *a. proposing appropriate treatments.
   b. formulating hypotheses.
   c. gathering data concerning a person's psychological state.
   d. drawing conclusions about a person's psychological state.

   Page: 96   Topic: Psychological Assessment

2. Dr. Nguyen is interviewing a new client. Although Dr. Nguyen will attempt to do all of the following in this first session, it is unlikely that she will be able to
   a. gather information about the client's history, life situation, personal relationships, and outlook for the future.
   *b. establish sufficient rapport with the client for the client to feel comfortable about revealing herself.
   c. gain information about the client from her general appearance, tone of voice, body posture, facial expressions, and eye contact.
   d. be attentive to the client's emotions and reflect those emotions back to the client in a nonjudgmental way.

   Page: 97   Topic: Clinical Interviews

3. Based on the research concerning "match" between interviewer and interviewee, which of the following therapist-client pairs would be anticipated to have the BEST outcome?
   a. Dr. Freud, a male therapist, and Anna, a woman who has recently been raped
   b. Dr. Anderson, an Anglo female therapist, and Maria, a Latina woman having marital problems
   *c. Dr. Park, an Asian male therapist, and Jae-Won, a Korean male who is having adjustment problems in college
   d. Dr. Fromm, an Anglo male therapist, and Dae, a depressed Asian male

   Page: 97   Topic: Clinical Interviews

4. Dr. Dreyer wants to learn about a client's current neurological and psychological functioning. In this process, Dr. Dreyer will look at the client's memory, sensation, activity level, mood, and clarity of thought. He is administering
   a. a structured interview.
   b. an unstructured interview.
   c. a psychometric examination.
   *d. a mental status examination.

   Page: 98   Topic: Structured Versus Unstructured Interviews

5. The mental status examination differs from the structured interview in that the former
    *a. permits clinicians the freedom to devise case-specific questions and pursue interesting leads as they arise.
    b. permits clinicians the freedom to devise case-specific questions, but does not encourage them to pursue interesting leads that may arise.
    c. sets out specific questions that guide the interview, but allows some flexibility in pursuing some leads if they seem especially important.
    d. requires that clinicians go through the questions one by one, without deviating from the interview protocol.

    Page: 98   Topic: Structured Versus Unstructured Interviews

6. Dr. Estim created a test to measure self-concept. Unfortunately, when he administered the instrument to a test sample, he realized that it measured social desirability instead. Dr. Estim's test was lacking in
    a. objectivity.
    *b. validity.
    c. reliability.
    d. clarity.

    Page: 99   Topic: Validity of Interviews

7. The modern era in psychological testing began with the work of
    a. Sigmund Freud.
    b. Charles Darwin.
    *c. Francis Galton.
    d. Alfred Binet.

    Page: 99   Topic: Intelligence Assessment

8. Alfred Binet was commissioned by the French government to develop a
    a. way to help children perform better in school.
    b. battery of tests to assess personality traits.
    c. test that could predict which children would benefit from placement in gifted programs.
    *d. test that could be used to predict which children would need special education.

    Page: 99   Topic: Binet's Test

9. Carlos has a mental age of 15 and a chronological age of 10. This would mean that
    *a. Carlos is above average in intelligence.
    b. Carlos is of average intelligence.
    c. Carlos is below average in intelligence.
    d. there was a problem with the test administration.

    Page: 99   Topic: Binet's Test

10. Wechsler's intelligence scales are popular for all of the following reasons EXCEPT:
    a. they have high reliability.
    *b. they are culturally unbiased.
    c. they have high validity.
    d. there are different forms for administration, depending on a person's age.

    Pages: 100–101   Topic: Wechsler's Tests

11. Tests using stimuli that elicit a wide range of different responses are called _____ tests.
    a. objective
    b. personality
    *c. projective
    d. subjective

    Page: 103   Topic: Projective Personality Tests

12. Mrs. Saks was given a series of psychological tests by her psychiatrist. The one she found most fascinating consisted of inkblots. This test is the
    a. Thematic Apperception Test.
    b. MMPI.
    c. Bender-Gestalt.
    *d. Rorschach test.

    Page: 103   Topic: Projective Personality Tests

13. The Rorschach inkblot test has been used to do all of the following EXCEPT
    *a. develop a specific diagnosis.
    b. bypass the ego's defenses.
    c. get people to talk.
    d. uncover repressed conflicts.

    Page: 104   Topic: Projective Personality Tests

14. As noted in the case of Danielle, a client's responding to noncentral aspects of the Rorschach cards would suggest
    a. depression.
    *b. an unwillingness to confront problems.
    c. overemphasis on achievement.
    d. suicidal tendencies.

    Page: 105   Topic: Document 3.6: Dr. Berg's Interpretation of One of Danielle's Rorschach Responses

15. Danielle was shown a series of cards and was asked by Dr. Berg, "Can you tell me who the people in this picture are, what is happening between them, what they are thinking or feeling, and what will happen in the future?" Which personality assessment was the clinician administering?
    a. the Bender-Gestalt
    b. the MMPI
    *c. the Thematic Apperception Test
    d. the Rorschach

    Page: 105   Topic: Projective Personality Tests

16. Why do clinicians remain committed to the use of projective techniques?
    a. Validation studies have shown them to be highly useful diagnostic measures.
    b. They offer a useful means of confirming diagnostic hypotheses.
    c. There has been relatively high agreement between experts' blind assessments and those of the treating clinicians.
    *d. When used as extensions of interviews, they provide useful ways to generate clinical hypotheses.

    Page: 107   Topic: Projective Tests: Current Status

17. Hathaway and McKinley combed psychology textbooks, novels, folk stories, anecdotes, and clinical case studies for self-descriptive statements to help them devise which personality test?
   *a.   the MMPI
    b.   the TAT
    c.   the Rorschach
    d.   word association

    Page: 107   Topic: Self-Report Tests

18. The most widely used clinical self-report test is the
    a.   CPI.
   *b.   MMPI.
    c.   Rorschach.
    d.   TAT.

    Page: 108   Topic: Self-Report Tests

19. Dr. Butler devised a new personality test and administered it to a representative sample of the general population so she could establish a set of "norms" from within the distribution of scores in the sample she studied. Then, people who take the test afterwards can be compared with this "norming" group. This illustrates the process of
    a.   reliability testing.
    b.   test validation.
   *c.   standardization.
    d.   test administration.

    Page: 108   Topic: Self-Report Tests

20. A criticism of the MMPI-2 is that
    a.   it omitted too many of the original questions from the MMPI.
    b.   it has not been tested sufficiently.
    c.   too many minority group members were included.
   *d.   the standardization sample was better educated than the population at large.

    Page: 108   Topic: Self-Report Tests

21. The first step in interpreting an MMPI protocol is to
   *a.   inspect its validity scales.
    b.   inspect its clinical scales.
    c.   look for peaks in the profile.
    d.   find any responses that may result from cultural differences.

    Page: 108   Topic: Self-Report Tests

22. How does the California Psychological Inventory (CPI) differ from the Minnesota Multiphasic Personality Test (MMPI)?
    a.   The CPI was designed specifically for people who live in California, taking into account their more casual approach to life.
   *b.   The CPI is intended to measure the dimensions of the normal personality, rather than the abnormal personality.
    c.   The CPI is designed to predict which children will require special education and counseling.
    d.   The CPI is a better predictor of clinical disorders, such as depression and schizophrenia, than the MMPI is.

    Page: 108   Topic: Self-Report Tests

23. Angela has been given a personality test with 21 sets of four-choice items, such as "I am not particularly discouraged about the future; I feel discouraged about the future; I feel I have nothing to look forward to; I feel that the future is hopeless and that things cannot improve." The therapist is probably trying to assess Angela's
   a. contact with reality.
   b. suicidal ideation.
   *c. depressive attributional style.
   d. achievement motivation.

   Page: 110   Topic: Self-Report Tests

24. All of the following are advantages of computerized tests EXCEPT:
   a. they are inexpensive.
   b. they can increase efficiency.
   c. they can produce routine reports.
   *d. they produce valid interpretations.

   Page: 111   Topic: Computerized Personality Tests

25. To detect subtle signs of disturbances of brain function, psychologists use
   *a. neuropsychological tests.
   b. MRIs.
   c. CAT scans.
   d. brain imaging techniques.

   Page: 111   Topic: Neuropsychological Assessment

26. Neuropsychological tests may be used to
   a. determine the cause of biologically based psychological problems.
   *b. localize the site of brain damage.
   c. provide clear images of the extent of brain damage.
   d. provide clear images of the location of brain damage.

   Page: 111   Topic: Localization of Brain Damage

27. Dr. Brewer is conducting a neurological assessment on Mr. Mahood. She has noted that he is having difficulty in language processing. This problem likely suggests damage to the
   a. sensory cortex.
   b. right hemisphere
   *c. left hemisphere.
   d. frontal lobes.

   Page: 113   Topic: Localization of Brain Damage

28. Dr. Martinez-Navarro is concerned that his client, Carlos, has neurological damage. Dr. Martinez-Navarro particularly wants to determine if there is damage to parts of the brain associated with higher order thinking skills. The neurological test uses 64 cards with different numbers, shapes, and colors, and Carlos is supposed to figure out, through trial and error, how the cards should be sorted. This test is the
   _____ Test.
   a. Bender-Gestalt
   b. Luria-Nebraska Neuropsychological Battery
   c. Wechsler Memory Scale–Third Edition
   *d. Wisconsin Card Sorting

   Page: 113   Topic: Localization of Brain Damage

29. Behavioral assessment is concerned with
    *a. describing the environmental conditions that elicit and maintain problem behaviors.
    b. identifying specific behaviors that appear to be problematic.
    c. devising specific techniques to eliminate problem behaviors.
    d. analyzing specific components of problem behaviors.

    Page: 114   Topic: Behavioral Assessment

30. Dr. Englebert uses an SORC analysis to conduct behavioral assessments of her clients. To obtain the necessary information for her SORC analyses, she would use all of the following EXCEPT
    a. interviews.
    *b. projective tests.
    c. self-report measures.
    d. direct observation.

    Page: 114   Topic: SORC Analysis

31. Angelica was seeing Dr. Humphreys for her behavior problems. Dr. Humphreys takes a behavioral approach to therapy, so we would expect her to elicit all of the following from Angelica EXCEPT
    a. the antecedents of Angelica's problem behaviors.
    b. the consequences of Angelica's problem behaviors.
    *c. personality traits that may be causing Angelica's problem behaviors.
    d. Angelica's thoughts in different situations.

    Page: 114   Topic: Self-Report Measures

32. Cash is being assessed for attention-deficit/hyperactivity disorder. His therapist, Dr. Rose, has noticed that Cash is well behaved and attentive when they are interacting with each other in her office. To get a better idea about Cash's typical behavior, Dr. Rose pays a visit to his school and observes him in his class activities. This is an example of _____ observation.
    a. participant
    b. clinic
    c. field
    *d. naturalistic

    Page: 114   Topic: Direct Observation of Behavior

33. The behavioral avoidance test measures
    *a. both severity of fear and treatment success.
    b. only severity of fear.
    c. techniques used for avoiding aversive situations.
    d. success at avoiding aversive situations.

    Page: 115   Topic: Direct Observation of Behavior

34. Self-monitoring is a
    a. proactive measure.
    *b. reactive measure.
    c. behavioral reduction technique.
    d. self-defeating treatment strategy.

    Page: 115   Topic: Direct Observation of Behavior

35. ABAB and multiple baseline designs are examples of _____ experiments.
    a. operant-conditioning
    b. classical-conditioning
    *c. single-subject
    d. target-behavior

    Page: 115   Topic: Ongoing Behavioral Assessment

36. L. S., who was sentenced to 20 years in prison for sexually molesting a young girl, is now being considered for parole. A condition of parole is that he no longer present a danger to society, particularly to young children. He is given a test in which he is shown photographs and films of young children to see if he becomes sexually aroused by these stimuli. He sexual arousal is then measured by using
    a. self-report.
    b. a polygraph.
    c. a biofeedback machine.
    *d. a penile plethysmograph.

    Page: 116   Topic: Psychophysiological Assessment

37. Avery had a problem that interfered with his job: fear of public speaking. His therapist decided they should record Avery's muscle tension while he was giving a speech, to provide him with information about when and how much he tenses and to determine how successful the treatment has been. The instrument used to record Avery's muscle tension is
    *a. an electromyograph.
    b. a polygraph.
    c. a plethysmograph.
    d. an electrocardiograph.

    Page: 116   Topic: Psychophysiological Assessment

38. The machine that is commonly known as a lie detector is technically called
    a. an electromyograph.
    *b. a polygraph.
    c. a plethysmograph.
    d. an electrocardiograph.

    Page: 116   Topic: Psychophysiological Assessment

39. Classifying disorders into diagnostic categories
    a. tells clinicians what caused a specific disorder.
    b. tells clinicians how to treat a specific disorder.
    *c. facilitates "shorthand" communication by clinicians.
    d. is an arbitrary way of dealing with symptomatic behaviors.

    Page: 117   Topic: Classifying Abnormal Behavior

40. After the American and French revolutions, as one of their first tasks, clinicians who worked in state hospitals set out to
    a. develop treatments for psychological disorders.
    b. separate the mentally ill from the physically ill.
    c. explain how and why different conditions develop.
    *d. classify their patients into diagnostic categories.

    Page: 117   Topic: The First *DSM*s

41. After World War II, the classification system for psychological disorders that was adopted around the world was
    a. the *International Statistical Classification of Diseases, Injuries, and Causes of Death (ICD).*
    b. the *Diagnostic and Statistical Manual (DSM).*
    c. both the *ICD* and the *DSM,* interchangeably.
    *d. the *ICD* in most of the world and the *DSM* in the United States.

    Page: 118   Topic: The First *DSMs*

42. The reason the American Psychiatric Association adopted the *DSM* rather than the *ICD* is that
    *a. the psychoanalysts who dominated the American Psychiatric Association rejected the *ICD*'s emphasis on physiological etiologies, stressing instead the role of traumatic experiences.
    b. members of the American Psychiatric Association wanted to separate themselves from the European influence inherent in adopting the *ICD.*
    c. members of the American Psychiatric Association, after reviewing the *ICD,* determined there were so many cultural differences between Europeans and Americans that the *ICD* would not be helpful in the United States.
    d. the panelists who wrote the *DSM* did so before the World Health Organization produced the *ICD,* and they chose not to convert to the *ICD* system.

    Page: 118   Topic: The First *DSMs*

43. The *DSM-II* category that referred to people whose psychological problems were not sufficiently severe to require hospitalization was
    a. reactions.
    *b. neuroses.
    c. psychoses.
    d. asymptomatic.

    Page: 118   Topic: The First *DSMs*

44. The *DSM-II* was criticized for many reasons. One of the most vocal critics, Thomas Szasz, criticized it on the grounds that
    a. diagnoses lack reliability.
    b. diagnoses lack validity.
    *c. diagnoses are social constructions.
    d. diagnostic labels may become self-fulfilling prophecies.

    Page: 118   Topic: Criticism I: Diagnoses Are Social Constructions

45. A problem related to the reliability of the diagnoses in the *DSM-II* involved
    a. inconsistency of the tests that were administered to determine what disorder a person had.
    b. use of the *DSM-II* by some clinicians while others used the *ICD.*
    c. a rift between psychoanalysts and psychologists in focusing on etiology and symptomatology.
    *d. disagreement among clinicians on diagnoses because the diagnoses were often stated in vague terms.

    Page: 118   Topic: Criticism II: Diagnoses Lack Reliability

46. Rosenhan's (1973) study using "pseudopatients" who were admitted to mental hospitals and diagnosed with psychological disorders underscores which criticism of diagnostic practices?
    *a. lack of diagnostic validity.
    b. overzealousness on the part of hospital admissions staff
    c. overreliance on social judgments
    d. lack of diagnostic reliability

    Page: 120   Topic: Criticism III: Diagnoses Lack Validity

47. Kate was diagnosed as bipolar. Thereafter, whatever she did was seen as pathological by her friends and family members. This was so even if someone considered "normal" engaged in behaviors similar to hers. This suggests that
   a. everyday behaviors may actually be symptomatic of a psychological disorder.
   *b. diagnostic labels may become self-fulfilling prophecies.
   c. Kate's diagnosis was in error.
   d. there is a lack of agreement on what constitutes abnormal behavior.

   Page: 120   Topic: Criticism IV: Diagnostic Labels May Become Self-Fulfilling Prophecies

48. A major impetus for revising the *DSM-II* was
   a. its lack of reliability.
   b. the public's outrage that "sane" people could be admitted to mental hospitals.
   *c. money.
   d. more information about psychopathology.

   Page: 121   Topic: Response to the Critics: *DSM-III* and *DSM-III-R*

49. Reasons for excluding the diagnosis of premenstrual dysphoric disorder (PMDD) from the *DSM-IV* included all of the following EXCEPT:
   a. it was seen as a form of the normal premenstrual syndrome that affects many women.
   b. including it would define normal female behavior as deviant.
   c. including it would stigmatize women and promote discrimination against them.
   *d. it did not meet the necessary criteria for inclusion.

   Page: 122   Topic: The *DSM-IV*

50. Diagnostic categories in the *DSM-IV* are based on
   *a. either etiology or symptomatology.
   b. etiology.
   c. symptomatology.
   d. nosology.

   Page: 122   Topic: The *DSM-IV*

51. The text states that, based on criteria in the *DSM-IV*, the "pseudopatients" in Rosenhan's study would not be diagnosed as schizophrenic today because
   a. they would instead be diagnosed with major depression.
   *b. they would not meet the specific criteria for a diagnosis.
   c. based on their individual histories, each would be diagnosed differently.
   d. the mental hospitals are now more sensitive to pseudopatients.

   Pages: 123–124   Topic: Specification of Diagnostic Criteria in the *DSM-IV*

52. A comparison between the *DSM-II* and the *DSM-IV* would suggest that
   a. there are fewer diagnostic categories in the *DSM-IV*.
   b. the *DSM-IV* has separated the neurotic disorders from the psychotic disorders.
   *c. diagnostic categories in the *DSM-IV* are more detailed.
   d. the *DSM-IV* provides treatment options for many of the disorders.

   Page: 124   Topic: Specification of Diagnostic Criteria in the *DSM-IV*

53. The *DSM-IV* uses five separate dimensions to provide different types of information about a person's diagnosis. This is called _____ diagnostic system.
   a. a five-axis
   b. an assessment
   c. a clarifying
   *d. a multiaxial

   Page: 124   Topic: Multiaxial Classification

54. The axis that considers how well a person is performing in psychological, social, and occupational areas is
   *a. Global Assessment of Functioning Scale
   b. Clinical Disorder(s)
   c. Personality Disorder(s)
   d. Psychosocial or Environmental Problems

   Page: 124   Topic: Multiaxial Classification

55. The multiaxial diagnosis of Danielle Wood indicated her current GAF to be 50. This would indicate that
   a. at the time of evaluation, she exhibited superior functioning in a wide range of activities.
   *b. at the time of evaluation, she exhibited moderate symptoms or moderate difficulty in her social or school functioning.
   c. at the time of evaluation, she exhibited some danger of hurting herself or others.
   d. for the year before her evaluation, she exhibited moderate symptoms or moderate difficulty in her social or school functioning.

   Pages: 125–126   Topic: Multiaxial Classification

56. Criticisms of the *DSM-IV* include all of the following EXCEPT:
   a. not all of its diagnostic categories are derived from research.
   b. it contains disorders with no known etiology.
   *c. it fails to recognize physical and social factors that may affect a person.
   d. the reliability of some of its diagnostic categories is too low.

   Page: 126   Topic: Diagnosis and Classification: Current Status

57. Dr. Winkler was concerned about becoming overwhelmed by too much information about her clients. To simplify the complex cognitive tasks involved in making diagnoses and to reduce her cognitive load, she relied on stereotyped cognitive strategies such as:
   a. mnemonics.
   b. cognitive templates.
   c. cognitive rules-of-thumb.
   *d. judgment heuristics.

   Page: 128   Topic: Bounded Rationality and Judgment Heuristics

58. Dr. Wapner has been called in to consult on a case in which the client may be potentially suicidal. Based on his experiences with similar clients, Dr. Wapner would use _____ to estimate the probability that this client may be suicidal.
   *a. an availability heuristic
   b. a representativeness heuristic
   c. framing
   d. a clinical judgment

   Page: 128   Topic: Availability Heuristic

59. St. Elegius Hospital's psychiatric department has recently installed a computer program to assist its mental health professionals in making "expert" decisions about patients' problems. This state-of-the-art program would be expected to do all of the following EXCEPT
   a. help structure problems.
   *b. be fast.
   c. suggest hypotheses.
   d. evaluate decisions.

   Page: 131   Topic: Decision Aids and Decision Analysis; Decision Aids: Current Status

60. Perhaps the most important objection to using a computer-based program for making diagnostic decisions about a client is that they
   a. have not been particularly accurate.
   b. require extensive data and are difficult to formulate.
   *c. diminish the importance of clincians and devalue patients.
   d. take too much time.

   Page: 131   Topic: Decision Aids: Current Status

TRUE-FALSE QUESTIONS

61. A test is reliable if it really measures what it is purported to measure. (F)
   Page: 99   Topic: Validity of Interviews

62. Over the past 100 years, it appears from scores on IQ tests that people seem to be getting smarter. (T)
   Page: 104   Topic: Highlight 3.1: Are People Getting Smarter?

63. Personality traits allow us to predict how a person will act in various situations. (F)
   Page: 103   Topic: Personality Assessment

64. Research with projective tests has shown them to provide disappointing results in terms of validity. (T)
   Pages: 106–107   Topic: Projective Tests: Current Status

65. Profiles generated by the MMPI and the MMPI-2 will always agree. (F)
   Page: 108   Topic: Self-Report Tests

66. Professional ethics require psychologists to use computerized reports cautiously. (T)
   Page: 111   Topic: Computerized Personality Tests

67. Tests designed for adults cannot be used with children unless they are modified to take developmental level into account. (T)
   Page: 114   Topic: Children and Brain Damage

68. Behavioral assessment is conducted at the first therapeutic session, and on an intermittent basis after the first assessment session. (F)
   Page: 114   Topic: Behavioral Assessment

69. There are times when ABAB (baseline/reversal) designs are not appropriate therapeutic techniques. (T)
   Page: 115   Topic: Ongoing Behavioral Assessment

70. Polygraphs have been found to be extremely valid general screening devices to measure honesty. (F)
   Page: 116   Topic: Psychophysiological Assessment

71. Psychological classifications are referred to as "diagnoses" because classification has its impetus in the medical context. (T)

    Page: 117   Topic: Classifying Abnormal Behavior

72. The diagnostic system used today for psychological disorders is based on the system devised by Emil Kraepelin. (T)

    Page: 117   Topic: The First *DSM*s

73. Given the same diagnostic skill and the same paradigmatic orientation, clinicians who have the same information about clients will consistently make the same diagnoses about these clients. (F)

    Page: 119   Topic: Critical Thinking About . . . 3.2: Clinical Agreement: Better Than Chance?

74. The *DSM-IV* and the *ICD-10* were written around the same time to ensure the comparability of research data collected in different countries and to maintain consistency between diagnostic systems. (T)

    Page: 121   Topic: The *DSM-IV*

75. The *DSM-IV* is a "political statement." (T)

    Page: 121   Topic: The *DSM-IV*

76. According to the diagnostic criteria of the *DSM-IV*, two people could receive the same diagnosis without sharing any symptoms. (T)

    Page: 124   Topic: Specification of Diagnostic Criteria in the *DSM-IV*

77. Long-term follow-ups have found that diagnoses cannot predict psychological problems later in life. (F)

    Pages: 127–128   Topic: Diagnosis and Classification: Current Status

78. A major breakthrough of the *DSM-IV* is its divergence from Kraepelin's categorical approach to classification. (F)

    Page: 127   Topic: Highlight 3.2: Are People More Than Simple Labels?

79. Researchers have not found statistically derived diagnoses to be more accurate than categorical diagnoses. (T)

    Page: 127   Topic: Highlight 3.2: Are People More Than Simple Labels?

80. Had Danielle's therapists used the subjective expected utility (SEU) approach to decision making, they could have effectively predicted her suicide. (F)

    Pages: 129–130   Topic: Decision Aids and Decision Analysis

SHORT-ANSWER QUESTIONS

81. What are the various uses of psychological assessments discussed in Chapter 3?

    They are mainly used to make diagnoses and plan treatments but are also used to help determine whether a person accused of a crime is competent to stand trial, whether a parent should be given custody of children in a divorce case, whether a person should be committed to or released from a hospital, whether a child requires special education, whether an applicant will be given a job; if administered both before and after treatment, they can indicate whether treatment was successful; and in some cases, assessments may reveal the etiology of psychological disorders.

    Page: 96   Topic: Introduction

82. Describe some of the problems inherent in achieving validity in a clinical interview.

Validity depends on the skill and experience of the interviewer. It can be compromised by clients' perceptions, their interpretations of psychologists' questions, and their background, education, and attitudes toward psychological problems and their situation. Interviewers may be biased, or they may emphasize information that is consistent with their preferred paradigm, discounting or ignoring inconsistencies.

Page: 99   Topic: Validity of Interviews

83. Discuss the common elements a clinician would look for in a client's responses when given the Thematic Apperception Test, and why these elements are important.

Clinicians typically search for consistent themes, such as aggression, guilt, dependence; they try to assess the adequacy of the hero (is the hero assertive, passive, successful, happy?) because people tend to "project" their own needs and feelings on the "hero" of their story; they try to judge how closely a person's story fits the picture and whether it seems reasonable (to assess whether the person has lost contact with reality).

Pages: 105–106   Topic: Projective Personality Tests

84. Explain the purpose of the four validity scales on the original MMPI.

High scores warn the examiner that the person's responses should not be accepted at face value. The L (Lie) Scale looks at common behaviors—a "no" response may reflect an attempt to appear in a socially desirable light. The F (Frequency) Scale contains bizarre statements that would be endorsed by someone trying to fake a psychiatric illness (but rarely endorsed by severely disturbed patients). The K (Correction) Scale, which measure defensiveness, may be used to correct clinical scales (a person with a high K Scale score and a moderately high score on a clinical scale is similar to a person with a low K Scale score and a high score on the clinical scale). Many omitted items ("Cannot Say" score) suggests indecisiveness (a sign of depression) or a reading problem, defensiveness, or uncooperativeness.

Page: 108   Topic: Self-Report Tests

85. Describe the five tests discussed in the text that are used to assess neurological problems.

The Luria-Nebraska Neuropsychological Battery and the Halstead-Reitan Battery of neuropsychological tests tap most information-processing stages; the Wechsler Memory Scale–Third Edition measures learning and memory; the Bender Visual Motor Gestalt Test consists of figures the client must copy to assess brain damage; the Wisconsin Card Sorting Test assesses signs of damage to those parts of the brain associated with higher order thinking skills.

Page: 113   Topic: Localization of Brain Damage

86. How is the behavioral interview similar to other types of clinical interviews, and how does it differ?

As in other interviews, questions in the behavioral interview cover physical health, history, current problems, family and peer relationships, and so on. However, instead of uncovering such issues as unconscious conflict, the behavioral interviewer seeks answers to specific "what" questions, such as "What behaviors, occurring in what situations, with what consequences are causing a problem?" For children, information may be solicited from parents or teachers rather than from the child.

Page: 114   Topic: Behavioral Interviewing

87. Explain the ABAB experimental design.

There are four phases. In the first, (A), baseline data are collected on the frequency and intensity of the problem behaviors; in the second, (B), treatment is introduced and changes are noted. To show that the treatment, rather than some other factor, was responsible for any improvement, the treatment is "reversed," or discontinued (A), but behavior continues to be monitored. If the problem behavior returns to baseline frequency, therapy is reinstated (B). If the positive changes noted earlier occur again, it is likely the treatment is responsible for those changes.

Page: 115   Topic: Ongoing Behavioral Assessment

88. What are the four criticisms presented in Chapter 3 of the early *DSM*s?

   Diagnoses are social constructions; diagnoses lack reliability; diagnoses lack validity; and diagnostic labels may become self-fulfilling prophecies.

   Pages: 118–121   Topic: The First *DSM*s

89. What were the three stages in development of the *DSM-IV?*

   First, work groups consisting of clinicians and researchers conducted systematic literature reviews to identify problems in the DSM-III-R diagnostic criteria; second, analyses were done of previously collected data; and third, field trials were conducted to assess the reliability of the diagnoses.

   Page: 121   Topic: The *DSM-IV*

90. Describe the five axes contained in the *DSM-IV.*

   Axis I contains a person's primary clinical diagnosis; Axis II describes any existing personality disorders; Axis III describes non-psychiatric medical conditions that may play a role in a person's problems; Axis IV indicates psychosocial or environmental problems that may affect the diagnosis, treatment, or prognosis of a mental disorder; and Axis V describes psychological, social, and occupational functioning on a hypothetical continuum from 1 (persistent danger of harm) to 100 (superior functioning).

   Pages: 124–125   Topic: Multiaxial Classification

91. Discuss the criticisms of the *DSM-IV.*

   Not all of its diagnostic categories are derived from research, it contains disorders with no known etiology, many of its diagnoses have no current treatment implications, the reliability of some of its diagnostic categories is still low, and its diagnostic labels carry stigmatizing connotations; also, it makes no clear distinction between normal and abnormal behavior.

   Page: 126   Topic: Diagnosis and Classification: Current Status

92. Explain the advantages and disadvantages of a dimensional approach to diagnosis and one way the text suggests for overcoming this problem.

   A dimensional approach would include all of a person's characteristics, which would provide a richer, more lifelike picture than is possible with a categorical diagnosis; but dimensional descriptions are more complex and harder to summarize, and there is no consensus about the appropriate dimensions to use. A factor analysis could be used to determine which dimensions "go together"; then patterns produced by dimensions that seem to co-vary could be given names, thus producing an alternative to traditional diagnoses.

   Page: 127   Topic: Highlight 3.2: Are People More Than Simple Labels?

93. Describe the two judgment heuristics that clinicians use to make clinical predictions and the potential problems with each.

   Availability heuristic: clinicians make predictions based on similar cases they have had; clinicians tend to overestimate disorders that receive a lot of journal coverage and underestimate those that get little coverage. Representativeness heuristic: clinicians base their judgments on how closely a specific client "represents" a stereotyped case; important information tends to be ignored.

   Pages: 128–129   Topics: Availability Heuristic; Representativeness Heuristic

94. What are the two important roles of expert-systems computer programs?

   They make diagnostic recommendations for solving problems, and they give advice; they also can serve a teaching role by identifying their reasoning process.

   Page: 129   Topic: Decision Aids and Decision Analysis

95. Describe the reasons clinicians have been slow to adopt decision aids.

   There is a belief that the research on clinical judgment has not been fair and that it has focused on less important aspects of clinical practice, such as diagnosis; the decision aids require a great deal of time in terms of data collection and analysis; decision rules are difficult to formulate; and most important, many feel that a reliance on "numbers" or external aids diminishes the importance of the clinician and devalues the individual patient.

   Pages: 129–130   Topic: Decision Aids: Current Status

ESSAY QUESTIONS

96. Your abnormal psychology professor has assigned your class the task of devising an effective test for predicting suicidal behaviors. In terms of developing this instrument, what technical concerns would you face?

   This will require a discussion of reliability and validity.

97. As you enter the cafeteria, you spot two friends from your abnormal psychology class. They are having a heated debate about what specific assessment devices are most useful to the clinician. One of your friends is a dyed-in-the-wool behaviorist, and the other is equally as committed to a psychoanalytic approach. They ask you for your opinion of all the assessment strategies you've learned in class. What would you tell them?

   This answer requires a discussion of interviews, intelligence tests, projective tests, self-report tests, neuropsychological assessments, and behavioral assessments, as well as comments as to which will provide what specific type of information.

98. Your Aunt Katie was diagnosed with bipolar disorder. Now it seems that whatever she says or does is interpreted within the framework of that diagnosis. Knowing that you are taking this class in abnormal psychology, she enlists your aid in talking to the family about both the benefits and detriments of "labeling." What could you tell your family?

   Diagnoses enhance communication by summarizing constellations of symptoms; they allow researchers to evaluate hypotheses on relatively homogeneous groups; and some may provide both etiological and therapeutic insights. However, they may be misleading, are potentially stigmatizing, give a great deal of power to mental health professionals, and set up the conditions for self-fulfilling prophecies, both by the person with the disorder and by that person's friends, relatives, and acquaintances.

99. Your study partners are having difficulty understanding the multiaxial diagnostic system used by the *DSM-IV*. They turn to you as the expert, to explain what it is, how many axes there are, what each one describes, and why such a system is even used. How would you explain it to them?

   This requires an explanation of the multiaxial diagnostic system as looking at several different dimensions; a discussion of the information provided by each of the five axes; and some insight into how providing additional information above and beyond a mere diagnosis can aid in understanding a client's problem.

100. After having been in your abnormal psychology class for several weeks, you are invited into a lab that has been set up for students in your department, as well as for the mental health professionals at the local hospital. You are curious to see that the computer seems not to have been used much. Based on what you've learned about making clinical judgments and using computer-based programs, what do you think this state-of-the-art computer could offer, and why do you think no one is using it?

   This requires a discussion of the diagnostic, treatment, and teaching potential of computer programs, together with the problems inherent in such programs.

CHAPTER 4
THE ANXIETY SPECTRUM: FROM EVERYDAY WORRY TO PANIC

MULTIPLE-CHOICE QUESTIONS

1. A common psychological disorder among soldiers during the Civil War was called
    *a. nostalgia.
    b. depression.
    c. shell shock.
    d. battle fatigue.

    Page: 136   Topic: A Casualty of War

2. The case study in the text about Dr. Carole Ballodi suggests that the origins of her anxiety symptoms appear to have come from her experiences of
    a. driving over a bridge.
    *b. tending to the wounded while under fire.
    c. having been sexually molested as a child.
    d. having a patient die in her office.

    Pages: 137–138   Topic: A Casualty of War

3. The case study in the text about Dr. Carole Ballodi states that she reacted to the sound of a helicopter as if she were in danger, even though no objective threat was present. The *DSM-IV* would refer to such an episode as
    a. a fear reaction.
    b. a panic disorder.
    *c. a panic attack.
    d. an alarm reaction.

    Page: 139   Topic: The Anxiety Spectrum

4. A panic attack is likely to include all of the following EXCEPT
    a. an abrupt and intense feeling of fear.
    b. physical symptoms of fear and panic.
    c. feelings of unreality or of being detached from oneself.
    *d. an objective danger or fear stimulus.

    Page: 139   Topic: Fear, Panic, and the Anxiety Disorders

5. According to Selye (1976), during the alarm reaction, all of the following are likely to occur when the sympathetic division of the autonomic nervous system is aroused EXCEPT:
    *a. blood supply to vessels near the skin increases.
    b. the amount of sugar in the blood increases.
    c. heart rate and respiration rate speed up.
    d. the supply of proteins that cause blood clotting increases.

    Page: 139   Topic: Fear, Panic, and the Anxiety Disorders

6. As Marabella walks into her classroom, she hears a strange, rattling sound. She turns toward the sound and sees a rattlesnake slithering toward her on the floor. Assuming Marabella is typical of most college students, her arousal state would be due to
   a. anxiety.
   *b. fear.
   c. a phobia.
   d. a panic attack.

   Page: 139   Topic: Fear, Panic, and the Anxiety Disorders

7. Shoshana fears leaving her home. She has set up a home-based business and has all of her supplies (as well as her groceries) delivered to her home. She has arranged her life so that she never has to go beyond the boundaries of her own yard. Based on this description, Shoshana has
   a. social phobia.
   b. generalized anxiety disorder.
   *c. agoraphobia.
   d. post-traumatic stress disorder.

   Page: 142   Topic: Table 4.2: The *DSM-IV* Anxiety Disorders

8. Armando fought in the Gulf War. He has flashbacks in which he continues to relive seeing his two best friends die in that conflict. Although he has a great deal of anxiety, he tells his therapist that emotionally he feels numb. Armando is suffering from
   a. social phobia.
   b. generalized anxiety disorder.
   c. agoraphobia.
   *d. post-traumatic stress disorder.

   Page: 142   Topic: Table 4.2: The *DSM-IV* Anxiety Disorders

9. The case study in the text about Dr. Carole Ballodi states that she is experiencing symptoms of several anxiety disorders. This is not unusual. Because panic and its related symptoms occur in practically all of the anxiety disorders, _____ is probably inevitable.
   *a. comorbidity
   b. coexistence
   c. correlation
   d. comingling

   Page: 142   Topic: Comorbidity and the Anxiety Disorders

10. According to Clarke and Watson (1991), anxiety and depression
    a. are rarely seen together.
    *b. may be variations in the expression of emotional distress.
    c. lead to physiological arousal.
    d. produce a negative mood.

    Page: 142   Topic: Comorbidity and the Anxiety Disorders

11. In the case study in the text about Dr. Carole Ballodi, Dr. Berg was called in to consult with Dr. Kahn to assess Carole and to
    a. evaluate her general medical status.
    b. determine whether drugs might be causing her problem.
    *c. help formulate a treatment plan.
    d. work with members of her family.

    Page: 143   Topic: Fears and Phobias

12. All of the following are true of phobias EXCEPT that
    a. they are persistent and irrational fears.
    b. more than 10% of the population has specific phobias.
    c. once they have started, phobias tend to last a lifetime unless they are treated.
    *d. they are evolutionarily adaptive.

    Page: 144   Topic: From Everyday Fears to Phobias

13. When Dorothy's youngest child, Richard, was 3 years old, he locked her in a closet. She banged on the door for a couple of hours until one of her daughters came home and let her out. Dorothy truly believed she was going to die in the closet, and ever since has refused to go into any confined space, including elevators and airplanes. Dorothy has
    *a. claustrophobia.
    b. acrophobia.
    c. cardiophobia.
    d. arachnophobia.

    Page: 146   Topic: From Everyday Fears to Phobias

14. Which of the following is the LEAST likely stimulus to be feared?
    *a. kittens
    b. dentists
    c. flying
    d. injury

    Page: 146   Topic: Determinants of Fears and Phobias

15. Which of the following is MOST likely to report a specific phobia?
    a. Arnold, an Anglo-American male.
    *b. Becka, an African American female.
    c. Carlotta, a Mexican American female.
    d. Denzell, an African American male.

    Page: 146   Topic: Cultural and Social Determinants

16. The findings that chickens fear hawks and most birds fear owls suggest that birds
    a. learn fear through classical conditioning.
    b. learn fear through modeling.
    *c. are born with those fears.
    d. are born with a predisposition to fear such stimuli, which develops as they mature.

    Page: 146   Topic: Hereditary Determinants

17. Assuming normal development, which child is MOST likely to exhibit a fear of strangers?
    a. 1-week-old Jeremiah
    b. 3-month-old Jenny
    c. 6-month-old Jasper
    *d. 8-month-old Jill

    Page: 147   Topic: Hereditary Determinants

18. The most common of all animal fears is the fear of
    *a. snakes.
    b. rats.
    c. mice.
    d. spiders.

    Page: 147   Topic: Highlight 4.1: Are We Born Fearing Snakes?

19. What indication is there that the fear of snakes is NOT due to the Freudian interpretation that snakes represent the penis?
    a. Watson demonstrated that the fear of snakes is classically conditioned.
    *b. Hebb demonstrated that chimpanzees also fear snakes, even if they have not been harmed by one.
    c. Skinner demonstrated that parents reinforce children's avoidance of snakes.
    d. Bandura demonstrated that children's fear of snakes is modeled on their parents' fears.

    Page: 147   Topic: Highlight 4.1: Are We Born Fearing Snakes?

20. Most psychologists believe that fears are learned through
    a. classical conditioning.
    b. operant conditioning.
    *c. both classical and operant conditioning.
    d. unconscious processes.

    Page: 148   Topic: Learning Experiences

21. Because Yeh was frightened of spiders, she refused to walk in the woods by her house. Even thinking about going into the woods (where spiders might be lurking) frightened her. By refusing to go into the woods, Yeh reduced her anxiety and _____ her fear.
    a. also reduced
    b. eliminated
    c. classically conditioned
    *d. strengthened

    Page: 148   Topic: Learning Experiences

22. Whether a person develops a specific phobia depends on all of the following EXCEPT the person's
    *a. sex.
    b. traumatic conditioning experiences.
    c. exposure to fearful models.
    d. genetic and cultural background.

    Page: 150   Topic: Learning Experiences

23. Subjects in the Schacter and Singer (1962) experiment interpreted their arousal as elation, anger, or fear depending on
    a. the amount of epinephrine they had been given.
    *b. their social context.
    c. their level of education.
    d. their personality traits.

    Page: 150   Topic: Cognitive Determinants

24. Which of the following students would be MORE concerned about fear of rejection than fear of performance?
    a. Pietra, a 16-year-old female student from Greece
    b. Jae-Won, an 18-year-old male student from Korea
    *c. Sequoia, a 17-year-old Native American male
    d. Momoko, a 17-year-old Japanese female

    Page: 151   Topic: From Performance Anxiety to Social Phobia

25. Performance anxiety is most commonly related to any of the following EXCEPT
   a. shyness.
   b. lack of confidence.
   c. self-consciousness.
   *d. traumatic experiences.

   Page: 151   Topic: From Performance Anxiety to Social Phobia

26. Social phobias usually develop in people who
   *a. are shy.
   b. have had a traumatic social experience.
   c. are elderly.
   d. have come to believe they are inadequate.

   Page: 152   Topic: Social Phobia

27. Sonia has been diagnosed by Dr. Breuer with avoidant personality disorder. With her symptoms, she is just as likely to be diagnosed by another clinician with which subtype of social phobia?
   a. performance
   *b. generalized
   c. limited interactional
   d. dependent

   Page: 153   Topic: Avoidant Personality Disorder

28. Albert has been plagued with a phobia of white, furry objects since infancy. When he finally decides to seek treatment for his problem, it is likely that his phobic reactions will be measured by all of the following EXCEPT
   a. self-report.
   b. behavioral observation.
   *c. objective testing.
   d. physiological measures.

   Page: 153   Topic: Measurement Comes First

29. Physiological measures of fear have the advantage of
   a. measuring a general tendency toward social anxiety.
   b. being less intrusive than other measures.
   c. using simple technology.
   *d. not being contaminated by social desirability.

   Page: 154   Topic: Physiological Measures

30. The first step in helping someone to overcome fears and phobias is to
   *a. establish a trusting relationship.
   b. assess the specific problem.
   c. assess the intensity and duration of the problem.
   d. consider the various treatment possibilities for the problem.

   Page: 154   Topic: Establish a Trusting Relationship

31. Which client is MOST likely to benefit from treatment?
   a. Mort, whose wife told him she would leave him if he didn't get therapy.
   *b. Manny, whose therapist told him what will happen in therapy and why.
   c. Millard, whose children said his behavior was potentially life-threatening.
   d. Max, who was told by the court that if he didn't get treatment, he would be sent to jail.

   Page: 154   Topic: Establish a Trusting Relationship

32. The three active ingredients described in the text that are necessary for treating clients with performance anxiety and social phobia are
    a. assessment, diagnosis, and empathy.
    b. accurate diagnosis, effective treatment plan, and appropriate prescription.
    *c. motivation, preparation, and exposure.
    d. observation, therapy, and follow-up.

    Pages: 154–155   Topic: Set Treatment Targets

33. Which therapeutic approach is most likely to include motivation, preparation, and exposure in treating social phobia and performance anxiety?
    a. humanistic
    b. behavior modification
    c. cognitive-behavior modification
    *d. all of the above

    Page: 155   Topic: Set Treatment Targets

34. Central to psychoanalytic theory is the idea that phobias are
    *a. symbolic representations of repressed impulses.
    b. ways to avoid unpleasant situations.
    c. techniques for indirectly expressing anger.
    d. problems that need to be treated before deeper problems can be addressed.

    Page: 156   Topic: Psychoanalytic and Humanistic Treatments

35. Cynthia has been seeing Dr. Franck for a phobia that is interfering with her ability to work. In an effort to help Cynthia overcome her phobia, Dr. Franck interprets Cynthia's dreams and free associations, and attempts to bring her unconscious thoughts into conscious awareness. Dr. Franck is using which approach?
    a. humanistic
    *b. psychoanalytic
    c. behavioral
    d. cognitive-behavioral

    Page: 156   Topic: Psychoanalytic and Humanistic Treatments

36. "What I hear you saying," said Dr. Carl to her client, "is that you feel as if you're going to embarrass yourself and sound foolish every time you get up to speak in public." Based on this statement, Dr. Carl is using which approach to therapy?
    a. behavioral
    b. cognitive-behavioral
    *c. humanistic
    d. psychoanalytic

    Page: 156   Topic: Psychoanalytic and Humanistic Treatments

37. Dr. Joseph is using systematic desensitization with a patient who suffers from performance anxiety. She will use all of the following steps EXCEPT
    a. relaxation training.
    b. constructing an anxiety hierarchy.
    c. gradual presentation of the anxiety hierarchy.
    *d. exposure to the most feared stimulus until the fear subsides.

    Page: 156   Topic: Behavioral Treatment

38. A phobia of _____ produces a SLOWING rather than an acceleration of a person's heart rate.
    *a. blood
    b. snakes
    c. public speaking
    d. needles
    Page: 157   Topic: Behavioral Treatment

39. Sarah attended a workshop in which a woman who had been debilitated by her inability to speak in public shared her feelings of anxiety and the steps she took to overcome her problem. Just listening to the speaker describe her experiences and strategies for overcoming her performance anxiety helped Sarah improve her performance. This demonstrates the power of which technique?
    a. systematic desensitization
    *b. modeling
    c. shaping
    d. skills training
    Page: 157   Topic: Behavioral Treatment

40. Dr. Baum works with clients who have performance anxiety. He teaches them about the role negative self-statements play in performance anxiety, then has them practice a set of more accurate self-statements, and finally, teaches them coping skills to help them deal with these situations. Which cognitive-behavioral technique is Dr. Baum using?
    a. cognitive restructuring
    b. rational-emotive
    *c. stress inoculation
    d. systematic desensitization
    Page: 158   Topic: Cognitive-Behavioral Treatment

41. John worked for the telephone company as a lineman, a job that required him to climb telephone poles. After falling off his roof while putting up holiday lights, he developed acrophobia, so that being up high created so much anxiety for him that he could not do his job. John decided to conquer his fear by climbing up a phone pole and staying there for 4 hours until his anxiety had totally subsided. This type of treatment is called
    *a. flooding.
    b. confrontational therapy.
    c. implosive therapy.
    d. self-exposure.
    Page: 157   Topic: Behavioral Treatment

42. The anxiolytic effects of _____ were discovered accidentally by researchers observing how various chemical compounds affect animal behavior.
    *a. chlordiazepoxide
    b. barbiturates
    c. propanediols
    d. diazepam
    Page: 159   Topic: Drug Treatment

43. The most common drug used today for anxiety is
    a. meprobamate (Miltown)
    *b. alprazolam (Xanax)
    c. fluoxetine (Prozac)
    d. diazepam (Valium)
    Page: 159   Topic: Drug Treatment

54

44. Side effects of benzodiazepines that have been substantiated by research include all of the following EXCEPT
    a. drowsiness.
    b. interference with cognitive functioning.
    *c. depression.
    d. drug dependence.

    Pages: 159–160   Topic: Drug Treatment

45. The personality assessment of Dr. Carole Ballodi in the text indicates that her score on trait anxiety was high. According to Dr. Berg, this would indicate
    a. that she views the world as a threatening place.
    b. a belief that the world harbors forces beyond her control.
    c. that she is currently feeling considerable anxiety about most aspects of her life.
    *d. a general tendency to react to major and minor challenges with fear and anxiety.

    Page: 160   Topic: Document 4.8: Excerpt from Dr. Berg's Psychological Assessment of Carole Ballodi

46. It's 7:30 p.m. and Jim is now half an hour late for his date with Anita. Anita worries that either he's been in an accident or he's going to stand her up, although he's never done that before. Worrying is not unusual for Anita: She seems to worry about everything, even when there appears to be nothing to worry about. She is constantly on edge, and even with weekly massage therapy, her muscles are always tense. Anita most likely suffers from
    *a. generalized anxiety disorder.
    b. panic attacks.
    c. panic disorder.
    d. obsessive-compulsive disorder.

    Page: 161   Topic: Generalized Anxiety Disorder

47. People with generalized anxiety disorder typically
    a. are diagnosed in clinics.
    *b. treat themselves with alcohol.
    c. are greater in number than people with phobias.
    d. receive a dual diagnosis if they have another disorder, such as post-traumatic stress disorder.

    Page: 162   Topic: Generalized Anxiety Disorder

48. Psychoanalysts attribute generalized anxiety disorder to
    a. a conflict between the id and the superego.
    b. a conflict between the ego and the superego.
    *c. a conflict between the ego and the id.
    d. an unresolved Oedipal conflict.

    Page: 162   Topic: Etiology of Generalized Anxiety Disorder

49. Jessica is a cognitive psychologist. She is most likely to believe that generalized anxiety disorder results from
    a. a conflict between the ego and the id.
    b. classical conditioning.
    c. a belief that no matter what we do, we cannot please the people around us.
    *d. fear of loss of control and helplessness.

    Page: 163   Topic: Etiology of Generalized Anxiety Disorder

50. One thing that psychoanalysts, behaviorists, and cognitive psychologists generally agree on with respect to generalized anxiety disorder is that it
    *a. develops only when there is a preexisting diathesis.
    b. has a genetic basis.
    c. must have some social trigger.
    d. generally is related to a biological component.

    Page: 163   Topic: Etiology of Generalized Anxiety Disorder

51. Freud's famous patient, the Rat Man, was suffering from
    a. a phobia of rodents.
    *b. obsessive-compulsive disorder.
    c. generalized anxiety disorder.
    d. agoraphobia.

    Page: 164   Topic: Obsessive-Compulsive Disorder

52. Mac washes his hands 100 times a day, no more, no less. Each time he washes them, he has a specific ritual that he uses. Mac's hand-washing is a form of
    a. anxiety production.
    b. obsession.
    *c. compulsion.
    d. anxiolysis.

    Page: 165   Topic: Obsessive-Compulsive Disorder

53. In most modern countries today, obsessions center around
    a. sin.
    b. toileting practices.
    c. religious practices.
    *d. cleaning or checking.

    Page: 165   Topic: Diagnostic Issues

54. Obsessive-compulsive disorder and obsessive-compulsive personality disorder are alike in that people suffering from both disorders typically
    *a. are overly orderly and clean.
    b. suffer from intrusive thoughts.
    c. feel compelled to perform rituals.
    d. derive pleasure from their behaviors.

    Pages: 165–166   Topic: Diagnostic Issues

55. D'Andre suffers from obsessive-compulsive disorder. We would expect his close relatives to have any of the following disorders EXCEPT
    a. obsessive compulsive personality disorder.
    *b. compulsive gambling.
    c. obsessional behavior patterns.
    d. depression.

    Page: 166   Topic: Diagnostic Issues

56. Drug studies suggest that obsessive-compulsive disorder is
    a. subject to the placebo effect.
    b. the result of harsh toilet training.
    *c. related to serotonin reuptake.
    d. related to excessive levels of dopamine.

    Page: 169   Topic: Biological Views

57. Dr. Conrad, a behavior therapist, finds that his major problem in treating obsessive-compulsive disorder is
    a. getting his clients to admit they have a problem.
    b. dealing with his clients' repetitive behaviors.
    c. his clients' lack of motivation.
    *d. getting his clients to complete the treatment.

    Page: 170   Topic: Treatment for Obsessive-Compulsive Disorder

58. Assuming treatment compliance, all of the following may be helpful for individuals with obsessive-compulsive disorder EXCEPT
    *a. use of antianxiety drugs.
    b. use of antidepressants.
    c. response prevention.
    d. thought-stopping.

    Page: 170   Topic: Treatment for Obsessive-Compulsive Disorder

59. Which of the following is NOT true of people with agoraphobia?
    a. They are predominantly female.
    *b. Most have a history of panic disorder.
    c. They begin by fearing only a few situations.
    d. They consider practically all situations outside the home to be potentially threatening.

    Page: 173   Topic: Diagnostic Issues

60. The research of Sanderson, Rapee, and Barlow (1989) suggests that _____ plays an important role in the etiology of panic attacks.
    a. carbon dioxide
    b. predictability
    *c. perception of control
    d. heredity

    Page: 174   Topic: The Mediating Effects of Cognition

61. Outcome studies on the effectiveness of treatment for panic attacks and agoraphobia have shown that
    a. drug therapy is the best way to begin, so the client can be relaxed enough to engage in other types of therapy.
    b. exposure therapy, without the use of drugs, has had the longest-lasting effects in terms of reducing panic attacks.
    c. those placed on a waiting list for therapy improved more than those who received drug therapy or cognitive-behavioral therapy.
    *d. cognitive-behavioral therapy, involving techniques such as cognitive restructuring, has shown the greatest improvement in long-lasting symptoms.

    Pages: 176–177   Topic: Psychological Treatment

62. Bourne (1990) and Craske and Barlow (1993) suggest a combination of all of the following techniques for treating panic disorder EXCEPT
    *a. drug therapy.
    b. cognitive restructuring.
    c. relaxation training.
    d. situational exposure.

    Pages: 176–177   Topic: Psychological Treatment

63. Wayne, a veteran of the Vietnam War, lost his brother and his best friend in the war and was then shunned by most people he encountered when he returned. Rhonda was raped by a man who broke into her home, blindfolded her, and threatened her with a knife held against her throat throughout the ordeal. Both Wayne and Rhonda suffer from an extreme anxiety response to traumatic, life-threatening events that were outside the range of normal human experience. They would both be diagnosed with
    a.   shell shock.
  *b.   post-traumatic stress disorder.
    c.   panic disorder.
    d.   obsessive-compulsive disorder.

    Page: 179   Topic: Post-Traumatic Stress Disorder

64. Symptoms of post-traumatic stress disorder differ for children and adults in that children
    a.   are more likely than adults to have flashbacks.
    b.   are less likely than adults to exhibit anxiety.
  *c.   are more likely than adults to show behavioral changes.
    d.   are more likely than adults to recover.

    Page: 180   Topic: Post-Traumatic Stress Disorder

65. The major buffering effect that would protect an individual from developing post-traumatic stress disorder is
    a.   psychological resilience.
    b.   genetic inheritance.
    c.   good physical health.
  *d.   a supportive environment.

    Page: 181   Topic: Vulnerability to Post-Traumatic Stress Disorder

66. The most common behavioral intervention for post-traumatic stress disorder is
  *a.   exposure.
    b.   systematic desensitization.
    c.   cognitive restructuring.
    d.   stress management training.

    Page: 182   Topic: Treatment of Post-Traumatic Stress Disorder

67. Dr. Hodges is treating a rape victim for her post-traumatic stress disorder. She asks her client to visualize the rape clearly, and the client then holds her head immobile as she follows the movements of a pencil Dr. Hodges holds. The treatment Dr. Hodges is using is called
    a.   hypnotism.
  *b.   eye movement desensitization.
    c.   cognitive restructuring.
    d.   visual imagery.

    Page: 182   Topic: Treatment of Post-Traumatic Stress Disorder

68. As stated in the text, the best treatment for post-traumatic stress disorder is
    a.   cognitive-behaviorism.
    b.   use of support groups.
  *c.   early intervention.
    d.   use of medication.

    Page: 182   Topic: Early Intervention and Prevention

69. When a researcher uses clients as their own control by switching subjects between groups, this is referred to as
   a. a stratified design.
   b. a controlled study.
   c. client selection.
   *d. a crossover design.

   Page: 184   Topic: Challenges in Assessing Treatment Outcome

TRUE-FALSE QUESTIONS

70. The theories and techniques developed to understand normal behavior are also applicable to psychological disorders. (T)

   Page: 139   Topic: Fear, Panic, and the Anxiety Disorders

71. Cued panic attacks, predisposed panic attacks, and uncued panic attacks have sufficiently different definitions that it is relatively easy to differentiate them from each other. (F)

   Page: 139   Topic: Fear, Panic, and the Anxiety Disorders

72. Panic attacks are common, especially among adolescents and college students. (T)

   Page: 139   Topic: Fear, Panic, and the Anxiety Disorders

73. The term used in the *DSM-IV* to describe distressing mental or behavioral symptoms that do not involve a serious break with reality is *neurosis.* (F)

   Page: 140   Topic: Fear, Panic, and the Anxiety Disorders

74. Anxiety is a feature of everyday life. (T)

   Page: 139   Topic: Fear, Panic, and the Anxiety Disorders

75. Fear is an important evolutionary adaptation. (T)

   Page: 144   Topic: From Everyday Fears to Phobias

76. The term *phobia* is derived from the Greek god Phobos, who was frightened of almost everything he encountered. (F)

   Page: 146   Topic: From Everyday Fears to Phobias

77. People who fear spiders report more aversive experiences with spiders than do people who do not fear spiders. (F)

   Page: 149   Topic: Learning Experiences

78. According to Bandura (1986), the real cause of fear is not the feared stimulus itself, but feelings of inadequacy in dealing with the challenge it presents. (T)

   Page: 150   Topic: Cognitive Determinants

79. The limited interactional subtype of social phobia is almost indistinguishable from avoidant personality disorder. (F)

   Page: 153   Topic: Social Phobia

80. When personality traits are extreme enough to produce deleterious effects on a person's life, the affected person is said to have a personality disorder. (T)

   Page: 153   Topic: Avoidant Personality Disorder

81. One reason that people have performance anxiety is that they overprepare for their performance. (F)

     Page: 155   Topic: Set Treatment Targets/Preparation

82. Empirical research suggests that the humanistic approach to dealing with anxiety disorders is the most effective. (F)

     Page: 156   Topic: Psychoanalytic and Humanistic Treatments

83. The rationale behind systematic desensitization is that a person cannot be both fearful and relaxed at the same time. (T)

     Page: 156   Topic: Behavioral Treatment

84. An extreme fear of snakes is very rare in children. (F)

     Page: 160   Topic: Document 4.8: Excerpt from Dr. Berg's Psychological Assessment of Carole Ballodi

85. The worry or associated somatic symptoms experienced by a person with generalized anxiety disorder cause significant impairment in social or occupational functioning or marked distress. (T)

     Page: 162   Topic: Table 4.8: Main *DSM-IV* Diagnostic Criteria for Generalized Anxiety Disorder

86. The specific nature of obsessions and compulsions varies across cultures. (T)

     Page: 165   Topic: Diagnostic Issues

87. Panic disorder is seen primarily in industrialized countries, rather than in less technologically advanced countries. (F)

     Page: 171   Topic: Panic Disorder and Agoraphobia

88. Both antihistamines and antidepressants are effective in reducing panic. (T)

     Page: 175   Topic: Treatment for Panic Disorder: Drug Treatment

89. Improvements on some measures may be statistically significant without necessarily being clinically significant. (T)

     Page: 185   Topic: Critical Thinking About . . . 4.1: Challenges in Assessing Treatment Outcome

SHORT-ANSWER QUESTIONS

90. How does fear differ from anxiety?

    Although both involve arousal of the sympathetic nervous system, fear serves the positive purpose of helping to mobilize the body's defenses in situations requiring fight or flight in response to an immediate threat. Anxiety has a less specific focus and does not serve such a purpose. Anxiety is characterized by apprehension about unpredictable dangers that lie in the future. However, some researchers suggest anxiety and fear are different emotions controlled by different parts of the central nervous system.

    Page: 139   Topic: Fear, Panic, and the Anxiety Disorders

91. What are the three categories of phobias in the *DSM-IV?*

    Specific phobias are fears of certain objects, organisms, and places; social phobia is an excessive concern about being evaluated by others; agoraphobia is the fear of being alone and unprotected in a threatening place.

    Page: 144   Topic: From Everyday Fears to Phobias

92. Describe the various theories addressing the belief that fear of snakes is (or is not) innate.

Watson believed that children are classically conditioned to fear snakes after they have been harmed by one; however, even children who have never encountered snakes may fear them. Psychoanalysts believe the fear of snakes is a symbolic representation of repressed sexual conflicts, with the snake representing the penis. However, Tau (1980) and Hebb (1946) demonstrated that even chimpanzees develop a fear of snakes by age 4, even if they have never been harmed by or even seen a snake. Rhesus monkeys in captivity do not seem to develop such a fear, however, which may negate the notion that this is an innate fear in human children. Ethics do not allow putting human children into captivity to test this!

Page: 147   Topic: Highlight 4.1: Are We Born Fearing Snakes?

93. What is the two-process theory of fear?

A phobia is acquired initially through classical conditioning. Over time, the person comes to avoid situations related to the one in which the original conditioning took place. Once it is generalized, the avoidance response fails to extinguish because avoiding feared objects reduces anxiety, which, in turn, instrumentally reinforces future avoidance.

Page: 148   Topic: Learning Experiences

94. Distinguish the three subtypes of social phobia, and state which personality disorder is related to social phobias.

Performance subtype: the phobic stimulus involves public performance of activities that can be engaged in comfortably if the individual is doing them while alone; limited interactional subtype: the phobic stimulus is restricted to one or two socially interactive situations, such as going out on dates or speaking to authority figures; generalized subtype: the phobic situation includes most social situations. The generalized subtype seems almost indistinguishable from avoidant personality disorder.

Page: 153   Topic: Social Phobia

95. What are the three active ingredients that the many different treatments share for dealing with performance anxiety and social phobia?

motivating people to change; ensuring that they prepare; exposing them to the feared stimulus

Page: 155   Topic: Set Treatment Targets

96. Describe the three parts of systematic desensitization and the rationale behind this treatment.

First: relaxation training; second: construction of an anxiety hierarchy in which fear-related images are arranged according to the degree of anxiety they elicit; third: graded presentation of hierarchy images while the person attempts to maintain a relaxed state. The rationale is that one cannot be both fearful and relaxed at the same time.

Page: 156   Topic: Behavioral Treatment

97. What are the five steps given in the text that individuals can take to overcome their fears.

confront your problem; critique your ideas; rehearse and prepare; learn to relax and develop coping skills; keep trying and get assistance

Page: 161   Topic: Highlight 4.2: Self-Help for Fears

98. Why do psychoanalysts believe that generalized anxiety disorder is a more serious condition than simple phobias?

By displacing anxiety onto a specific object, phobias help to lift anxiety. Phobic people need only to avoid the feared object to avoid the anxiety; people with generalized anxiety disorder have a more difficult time containing their anxiety because its source is within themselves and they carry it around wherever they go.

Page: 162   Topic: Etiology of Generalized Anxiety Disorder

99. Describe the person who is most susceptible to obsessive-compulsive disorder, in terms of gender, age, and life events. What impact does culture have on this disorder?

OCD affects between 2 and 3% of the population at some time in their lives, females more often than males; it generally first appears in late adolescence or early adulthood, often in conjunction with some significant life event. The specific nature of obsessions and compulsions changes from time to time and place to place, reflecting changes in the dominant culture.

Pages: 165–166 Topics: Diagnostic Issues; Highlight 4.3: Cultural Influences on Obsessive-Compulsive Symptoms

100. Explain the process by which panic attacks lead to agoraphobia.

If the initial attack, which may come on without warning, is followed by further attacks, the person comes to associate panic attacks with the situations in which they occur and, fearing further attacks, to avoid these situations. Over time, the attacks occur in other situations, which must also be avoided. As the number of situations to be avoided increases, the person's movements become increasingly restricted. This eventually gives rise to agoraphobia.

Page: 171 Topic: Panic Disorder and Agoraphobia

101. Explain the connection between panic attacks and carbon dioxide.

Without our conscious awareness, our respiratory system extracts oxygen from the atmosphere and excretes carbon dioxide. As long as the amount of carbon dioxide in our bloodstream stays within certain limits, our breathing is steady and effortless; but if the amount becomes too low, we begin to breathe rapidly, which can develop into hyperventilation. Because panic attacks sometimes begin with a feeling of suffocation followed by hyperventilation, some researchers hypothesize that panic attacks are triggered by abnormally low levels of carbon dioxide—or by an oversensitive internal monitoring mechanism that misjudges normal levels as too low.

Pages: 173–174 Topic: Carbon Dioxide–Induced Panic Attacks

102. Discuss the two methodological problems presented in the text concerning the connection between mitral valve prolapse and panic attacks.

First: diagnosing mitral valve prolapse from nonintrusive tests, such as electrocardiograms, is difficult, and experts often disagree. Second: the experimenters who were interpreting the EKGs usually knew which subjects suffered from panic disorder; thus, they may have been biased toward diagnosing prolapse in the panic disorder group, even when the findings were equivocal.

Page: 174 Topic: Mitral Valve Prolapse

103. What is the focus of most psychological treatments for panic disorder?

They are aimed at one or more of the variables that contribute to the fear of fear cycle: preoccupation with internal bodily states, excessive physiological responsiveness to threat, faulty cognitive appraisals, or the quickly spiraling loss of control.

Pages: 176–177 Topic: Treatment for Panic Disorder: Psychological Treatment

104. List the seven problems discussed in the chapter that are faced by therapy researchers.

client selection; biases; outcome criteria; prospective versus historical controls; stratified designs; crossover design; clinical versus statistical significance

Page: 184 Topic: Challenges in Assessing Treatment Outcome

ESSAY QUESTIONS

105. You come home late one evening to find your roommate hiding in a corner, shaking and sweating. He tells you that while studying, he saw a rat run across the floor, and ever since he was a young child, he's been frightened of rats, just as his mother used to be. He says that he believes everyone is afraid of rats and would probably react the same way he did. What can you tell him about the differences between fear and phobias?

    Explore the complex interaction of heredity, developmental stage, traumatic experiences, cultural norms, and instrumental learning; how some fears are more common than others; and the differences between fear and phobias in terms of reasonableness of response.

106. As you come into the student union, you notice three of your friends drinking coffee and having a heated argument about which type of therapy works best for the anxiety disorders. One believes psychoanalysis gets at the root of the problem, the second says that drug therapy deals with the underlying bases of these disorders, and the third says that the cognitive-behavioral approach is the one that has the best results in the long run. They turn to you for your opinion. How would you respond?

    Discuss the unconscious conflicts of the psychoanalytic approach, the notion that the disorder is merely symbolic of the underlying problem, the rationale for the biological approach in terms of etiology of anxiety disorders, and the cognitive-behavioral perspective on the etiology of the anxiety disorders. Then discuss the techniques used for each and what the outcome research says about effectiveness.

107. It's 2:00 a.m. and your mother comes into your room and tells you it's time to stop studying and get some sleep. You tell her it's important for you to study so that you can maintain your 4.0 GPA. She tells you she thinks you need to see a therapist because anyone who studies so much and feels it is so important to get straight A's must have obsessive-compulsive disorder, or at the very least obsessive-compulsive personality disorder. Explain to her the differences between obsessive-compulsive disorder, obsessive-compulsive personality disorder, obsessive behavior, and just being a good student.

    Discuss the diagnostic issues related to each of these three disorders, including the intrusive thoughts and ritualistic behaviors of OCD; the milder nature of obsessive-compulsive personality disorder, with its lack of obsessive thoughts and compulsive behaviors; how both differ from so-called compulsive behaviors such as gambling; and how hard work and studying are not abnormal behaviors for students and are necessary for getting good grades.

108. On the first day of class, your professor says that during the last week of the term, everyone will have to give individual presentations. You can start to feel your mouth become dry, your skin develop goose bumps, and your stomach turn, as you begin to sweat and feel nauseated. You need this class to graduate, so you know you can't drop it. What steps can you take that will help you get through this project?

    Use the five steps given for self-help for fears: confront your problem, critique your ideas, rehearse and prepare, learn to relax and develop coping skills, and keep trying and get assistance.

109. When you come home from classes one evening, you learn that a neighbor has been taken to a mental health facility because he was suffering from extreme anxiety. He was having flashbacks and suddenly started talking strangely and became highly agitated and aggressive. When you visit his mother, she tells you he's never been quite the same since he came back from the Gulf War. She says the medics who took him away said he was suffering from post-traumatic stress disorder, but she doesn't know what that means. How would you explain the disorder to her, and what could you tell her about the types of treatment that will probably be most helpful to her son?

    Explain the symptoms, etiology, treatments, and importance of a support system.

CHAPTER 5
EFFECTS OF STRESS ON HEALTH AND DISEASE

MULTIPLE-CHOICE QUESTIONS

1. In the case study of William Cole, it was noted that the _____ is particularly affected by diabetes because glucose is the only nutrient it can metabolize.
    *a. brain
    b. pancreas
    c. liver
    d. spleen

    Page: 194   Topic: Living With Chronic Illness: William Cole's Story

2. The third leading cause of death in the United States is
    a. heart disease.
    *b. Type 1 diabetes.
    c. Type 2 diabetes
    d. vehicular accidents.

    Page: 195   Topic: Living With Chronic Illness: William Cole's Story

3. Psychosomatic illnesses are illnesses that are
    a. not real.
    b. psychological, not physical.
    *c. physical, but psychological factors play a role in their etiology.
    d. physical illnesses that affect a person's psychological well-being.

    Page: 195   Topic: Psychosomatic Versus Physical Illness: A Dubious Distinction

4. As the text notes, peptic ulcers are the result of a bacterial infection, caused by *Helicobacter pylori,* which thrives in the acidic environment produced by stressful conditions. This is an example of which model of psychopathology?
    a. psychoanalytic
    b. behavioral
    c. behavioral-cognitive
    *d. diathesis-stress

    Page: 195   Topic: Psychosomatic Versus Physical Illness: A Dubious Distinction

5. The goal of behavioral medicine that is becoming increasingly important now that many diseases have been eradicated is learning how psychological factors
    *a. affect health-related behavior.
    b. determine compliance with medical treatment.
    c. alter the course of an illness.
    d. make people susceptible (or resistant) to illness.

    Page: 195   Topic: Psychosomatic Versus Physical Illness: A Dubious Distinction

6. With respect to the interaction between psychological and physiological factors, which is MOST true?
   a. Psychological factors can cause a medical condition.
   *b. Psychological factors can cause or exacerbate a medical condition, and physiological factors can produce or exacerbate psychological problems.
   c. Physiological factors can produce or exacerbate psychological problems.
   d. Psychological factors and physiological factors are separate and largely noninteractive.

   Page: 195   Topic: Psychosomatic Versus Physical Illness: A Dubious Distinction

7. As indicated in the case study of William Cole, the first step in managing William's blood sugar levels is to
   a. inject insulin before breakfast and dinner.
   b. balance his insulin and food intake.
   *c. monitor his blood sugar levels through accurate blood testing.
   d. monitor his insulin levels through urinalysis.

   Page: 197   Topic: Managing a Chronic Illness

8. Which of the following would argue that the mind and the body are separate entities?
   a. Hippocrates
   b. Aristotle
   c. Sigmund Freud
   *d. René Descartes.

   Page: 198   Topic: Origins

9. Dr. Camus is a medical scientist who was heavily influenced by Descartes. Knowing that Dr. Camus subscribes to Descartes's philosophy, we would expect him to focus his efforts on
   *a. uncovering disease-causing agents such as bacteria.
   b. determining the psychological factors that underlie disease.
   c. looking for the interactions between the physiological and the psychological factors of disease.
   d. seeking a way to eradicate disease by providing individuals with the maximum amount of freedom.

   Page: 198   Topic: Origins

10. Madeline, a young woman of the 19th century, had symptoms of fatigue, aches and pains, sore throat, and low-grade fever. Her doctor would most likely have diagnosed her with
    a. melancholia.
    *b. neurasthenia.
    c. chronic fatigue syndrome.
    d. ague.

    Page: 198   Topic: Psychoanalytic Views on the Physical Symptoms of Hysteria

11. Anna passed through various phases in her treatment, including loss of the use of her right hand, functional blindness, and false pregnancy. There was no neurological or physiological basis for any of these problems. Freud would have called the problem
    a. neurasthenia.
    b. psychosomatic disorders.
    *c. conversion hysteria.
    d. malingering.

    Page: 199   Topic: Psychoanalytic Views on the Physical Symptoms of Hysteria

12. Walter Cannon (1939) believed that organisms faced with a threatening stimulus mobilize their physiological resources to combat or escape the threat. He referred to this as the
    a. fight or flight response.
    b. general adaptation syndrome.
    c. alarm reaction.
    *d. emergency reaction.

    Page: 199   Topic: Psychosomatic Medicine

13. After studying the effects of prolonged stress on health, Cannon concluded that
    *a. voodoo deaths are caused by the intense autonomic reactions produced by fear.
    b. soldiers who develop ailments such as peptic ulcers and coronary heart disease are trying to get out of the service.
    c. early childhood experiences are a major determining factor in whether prolonged stress can lead to physical illness.
    d. stories about people who die of fright or sadness are folk myths.

    Page: 200   Topic: Psychosomatic Medicine

14. Khalil has a peptic ulcer. If a researcher were using specificity theory, as elaborated by Franz Alexander, he or she would attribute the ulcer to:
    a. sadness and repressed crying.
    *b. conflict over dependency needs.
    c. repression of hostile impulses.
    d. avoidance of overt expressions of aggression.

    Page: 200   Topic: Specificity Theory

15. Arthur is impatient, competitive, always on the go, ambitious, and a workaholic. According to the research of Friedman and Rosenman (1974), what type of personality does Arthur have?
    a. aggressive
    b. overbearing
    *c. Type A
    d. Type B

    Pages: 202–203   Topic: Critical Thinking About . . . 5.1: The Rise and Fall (and Rise) of the Type A Behavior Pattern

16. Which aspects of the Type A personality have been found to be correlated with coronary heart disease?
    a. all of them
    b. always being on the go, being ambitious, and being a workaholic
    c. aggressiveness and competitiveness
    *d. hostility, cynicism, and anger

    Page: 203   Topic: Critical Thinking About . . . 5.1: The Rise and Fall (and Rise) of the Type A Behavior Pattern

17. During the _____ stage of the general adaptation syndrome (GAS), the organism uses its physiological resources to minimize tissue damage.
    a. alarm
    b. emergency
    *c. resistance
    d. exhaustion

    Page: 201   Topic: Nonspecific Stress Theory

18. Which of the following is NOT a stressor?
    a. divorce
    b. getting fired
    c. winning the lottery
    *d. They are all stressors.

    Page: 203   Topic: Nonspecific Stress Theory

19. Malcolm's family moved to a new town when his father got a promotion and a transfer. Malcolm has always been emotionally immature and lagged behind his classmates in social skills. His parents are concerned that he will be unprepared to enter his new high school, which will require him to be more independent and autonomous. This describes
    *a. transitional stress.
    b. acculturative stress.
    c. specific stress.
    d. nonspecific stress.

    Page: 205   Topic: Psychosocial Development

20. Hyun-Joo came to the United States to study computer information systems. She got her bachelor's degree in computers from a Korean university but is afraid she won't succeed in her studies here because she is having difficulty understanding her professors and classmates, and they have difficulty understanding her. Living away from her family and having made few friends here, she feels isolated and incompetent. Hyun-Joo is experiencing _____ stress.
    a. transitional
    *b. acculturative
    c. specific
    d. nonspecific

    Page: 206   Topic: Cultural Conflict

21. Thomas Holmes determined that
    a. it is primarily negative life events, like the death of a loved one, that produce stress.
    b. it is primarily positive life events, like getting married, that produce stress.
    *c. both positive and negative life events can produce stress.
    d. it is not the life events, but how we handle them that produces stress.

    Page: 207   Topic: Important Life Events

22. The Life Changes Scale measures
    a. the degree of stress a person experiences from life events.
    b. the number of stressful events in a person's life.
    c. how well a person can adjust to stressful events.
    *d. the amount of readjustment an event requires.

    Page: 207   Topic: Important Life Events

23. Mauricio added up his life-change units over the past year and was surprised to see that they totaled 320. What would this score suggest?
    *a. Mauricio's score is high, so he has a strong chance of becoming ill.
    b. Mauricio's score is high, so he will soon become ill.
    c. Mauricio's score is average, so he has a moderate chance of becoming ill.
    d. Mauricio's score is low, so it is unlikely he will become ill.

    Page: 207   Topic: Important Life Events

24. All of the following make it difficult to interpret life-stress studies EXCEPT:
    a. life-stress research is typically retrospective.
    *b. life-stress researchers assume that bad events produce more stress than good events.
    c. individuals may appraise life changes in different ways.
    d. social and ethnic groups may differ in their appraisals of life events.

    Page: 210   Topic: Critical Thinking About . . . 5.2: Interpreting Life-Stress Research

25. Who is most likely to experience the greatest amount of stress?
    a. Eduardo, a 62-year-old Hispanic male, who plans to travel around North America once he retires next month.
    b. Samantha, a 25-year-old White female, who just won the lottery.
    *c. Hiroki, a 30-year-old Japanese male, who just got a ticket for jaywalking.
    d. Gerry, a 30-year-old White male, who just got a ticket for jaywalking.

    Page: 211   Topic: Critical Thinking About . . . 5.2: Interpreting Life-Stress Research

26. Kanner and colleagues (1981), in constructing the Hassles and Uplifts Scales, believed that
    a. hassles and uplifts both cause about the same amount of stress, depending on the specific event involved.
    b. hassles cause more stress than uplifts, but both create some stress.
    c. uplifts, surprisingly, can cause more stress than hassles.
    *d. uplifts have the power to counteract hassles.

    Page: 209   Topic: Everyday Hassles

27. According to the current stress research, stress can be produced by all of the following EXCEPT
    *a. uplifting life events.
    b. cultural conflict.
    c. everyday hassles.
    d. chronic illness.

    Pages: 204–209   Topic: Sources of Stress

28. Individuals who cope well with chronic pain typically have all of the following EXCEPT
    a. an optimistic personality.
    *b. a good education.
    c. good support networks.
    d. perception of control over their lives.

    Page: 211   Topic: Chronic Pain and Headaches

29. Recent research on headaches indicates that
    a. tension headaches result from tense muscles in the neck and head.
    b. tension headaches result from contraction and dilation of blood vessels in the head.
    *c. tension headaches and migraine headaches result from contraction and dilation of blood vessels in the head.
    d. tension headaches and migraine headaches result from tense muscles in the neck and head.

    Page: 212   Topic: Chronic Pain and Headaches

30. Some evidence suggests that people who cope well with pain
    a. metabolize opiates better than those who do not cope well with pain.
    b. are less likely to use opiates than those who do not cope well with pain.
    c. produce lower levels of endogenous opioids than those who do not cope well with pain.
    *d. produce higher levels of endogenous opioids than those who do not cope well with pain.

    Page: 212   Topic: Chronic Pain and Headaches

31. The body's response to stress differs for those with and without diabetes in that
    *a. once the stressor is removed, blood sugar levels that provided energy to mobilize the body's defenses return to normal in those without diabetes, but remain high in those who are diabetic.
    b. once the stressor is removed, blood sugar levels that provided energy to mobilize the body's defenses return to normal in those without diabetes, but increase in those who are diabetic.
    c. due to defective functioning of the pancreas, those with diabetes are unable to produce the high levels of sugar required to mobilize the body's defenses.
    d. due to an insufficient amount of insulin, those with diabetes produce excessive levels of sugar.

    Page: 212   Topic: Direct Physiological Effects of Stress

32. It is believed that stress leads to cardiac arrest and stroke by
    a. reducing inflammation and inhibiting pain.
    *b. weakening neurons in the hippocampus.
    c. producing an overabundance of proteins.
    d. producing hormones that turn off the stress response.

    Page: 212   Topic: Direct Physiological Effects of Stress

33. The branch of physiological psychology that studies the interactions among behavior, neurological and endocrine function, and the immune process is referred to as
    a. psychophysiology.
    b. neuroendocrinology.
    *c. psychoneuroimmunology.
    d. interactive psychoimmunology.

    Page: 212   Topic: Stress and the Immune System

34. The main organ of the body's immune system is the _____ system.
    a. endocrine
    b. alimentary
    c. respiratory
    *d. lymphatic

    Page: 213   Topic: Stress and the Immune System

35. Foreign invaders, such as bacteria, that make it past the body's first line of defense (the skin and mucous membranes) are attacked directly by the
    *a. T cells.
    b. B cells.
    c. natural killer cells.
    d. antigens.

    Page: 213   Topic: Stress and the Immune System

36. The corticosteroids and endorphins produced during the general adaptation syndrome (GAS) appear to decrease the effectiveness of
    a. antigens.
    *b. natural killer cells.
    c. T cells.
    d. B cells.

    Page: 263   Topic: Stress and the Immune System

37. An individual's health may be affected in the event that stress interferes with any of the following cognitive processes EXCEPT
    a. memory.
    b. judgment.
    *c. language.
    d. motivation.

    Page: 214   Topic: Indirect Effects of Stress on Health

38. On a whaling voyage, Captain Ahab and his crew found themselves in the worst storm any of them had ever experienced. It was so bad that the men had to tie themselves to the ship's masts to keep from being swept overboard. Captain Ahab, however, had sworn not to return to port until he had caught the great white whale. Being aware of the research on stress and cognition, we would expect that Captain Ahab would
    a. cautiously consider the needs of his crew.
    b. meet with his first mate to determine the safest procedures to follow.
    c. check his sailing manuals and equipment to plan the safest strategy.
    *d. order his men to pursue the great white whale despite the danger involved.

    Page: 215   Topic: Effects of Stress on Cognition

39. Pearl, who has diabetes, hates her job. She feels the other secretary is constantly trying to sabotage her and make her look bad. She long ago gave up on the idea of getting married and, for the past 30 years, has lived with her older sister, with whom she constantly argues. Based on the research concerning the effects of stress on motivation, we would suspect the reasons that Pearl frequently forgets to give herself insulin injections and often sneaks ice cream and other sweets include all of the following EXCEPT
    *a. her desire to die.
    b. a desire to punish herself.
    c. frustration.
    d. loneliness.

    Page: 215   Topic: Effects of Stress on Motivation

40. The most important factor that has been identified to predict compliance with treatment regimen for chronic illness is
    a. warm doctor-patient relationships.
    *b. the way in which people appraise the stress produced by illness.
    c. clear instructions for administration of medication.
    d. concern for one's health.

    Page: 216   Topic: Factors That Modify the Effects of Stress

41. The text discusses how appraisal of life events results in all of the following types of responses EXCEPT
    a. emotional
    b. physiological
    *c. spiritual
    d. behavioral

    Pages: 216–217   Topic: Appraisals

42. Emily has just received a letter advising her that she did not qualify for a scholarship that would have paid the entire cost of her tuition and books. Upon reading the letter, she assesses how this will affect her. Emily is engaging in
    a. rumination.
    b. rational appraisal.
    c. secondary appraisal.
    *d. primary appraisal.

    Page: 216   Topic: Appraisals

43. Having been notified that she will not receive a scholarship that would have paid for the entire cost of her tuition and books, Emily tries to decide what she will now have to do to meet these expenses. Emily is engaging in

    *a. secondary appraisal.
    b. primary appraisal.
    c. rumination.
    d. rational appraisal.

    Page: 216   Topic: Appraisals

44. Our response to stress is always based on our personal _____ external events.

    a. sensations about
    *b. perceptions of
    c. reactions to
    d. rationalizations about

    Page: 216   Topic: Appraisals

45. Scarlet has just been evicted, and her car is about to be repossessed by the bank. Her boyfriend tells her he is going to leave her because he can no longer handle the way she deals with her problems. Scarlet replies, "I'll worry about it tomorrow." According to Lazarus, Scarlet is using _____ coping.

    a. rational
    b. problem-focused
    *c. emotion-focused
    d. compulsive

    Page: 217   Topic: Appraisals

46. Rhett, who works full time, has final exams coming up in each of his six classes. His mother's birthday falls right in the middle of finals week, and he knows she will be disappointed if he doesn't celebrate it with her. Rhett decides the best way to keep his boss satisfied, his mother happy, and his grades up is to make a plan that will allow him enough time for work, school, studying, eating/sleeping, and family. Rhett is using which type of coping?

    a. rational
    *b. problem-focused
    c. emotion-focused
    d. compulsive

    Page: 217   Topic: Appraisals

47. In studying families who have a child with diabetes, Gustafsson (1987) found that

    a. there was little relationship between family harmony or conflict and control of blood sugar.
    b. it was difficult to make any determination about the relationship between family harmony or conflict and control of blood sugar due to the unreliability of self-report.
    c. contrary to the initial hypothesis, family harmony was a stronger predictor of poor control of blood sugar than was conflict.
    *d. conflicts during decision making were found to be related to poor control of blood sugar.

    Page: 218   Topic: Social Support

48. Hosea is a senior in high school. He has had diabetes since he was 12 years old. Based on the research concerning chronic illness, we would expect which source of social support to be most important for Hosea in controlling his diabetes?
   *a. friends
   b. parents
   c. siblings
   d. high school counselor

   Page: 218   Topic: Social Support

49. All of the following are characteristics of hardy people EXCEPT:
   a. they are committed to their work.
   *b. they believe events in their lives are controlled by outside forces.
   c. they view change as a challenge and an opportunity to grow.
   d. they address problems in a positive way.

   Page: 219   Topic: Hardiness

50. Although at present there is no clear link between stress and cancer, animal research suggests that link to be
   a. temperament.
   b. genetic.
   *c. immune suppression.
   d. hardiness.

   Pages: 220–221   Topic: Highlight 5.2: Personality, Stress, and Cancer

51. Dorothy no longer wants to live alone. Even though her children and her sister live nearby, she gets frightened at night and worries that she may fall and no one will be there to help her. After talking about it with her children, she chooses to live in an extended-care facility. We could expect Dorothy to live longer and to be healthier than those who are in nursing homes without their consent due to which factor of locus of control?
   a. utility
   b. predictability
   c. familiarity
   *d. controllability

   Pages: 221–222   Topic: Locus of Control

52. Robert has AIDS. He exercises every day, eats a healthy diet, and takes his medication as prescribed. Although his friend Anthony has noticed that Robert appears to be getting thinner and weaker, Robert tells him, "If I stick to the regimen, I'll be all right." This demonstrates which health belief?
   *a. the benefits of compliance
   b. susceptibility
   c. severity
   d. the costs of compliance

   Page: 222   Topic: Health Beliefs and Attributions

53. Looking at specific health beliefs, Brownlee-Duffeck and colleagues (1987) found that
   a. adherence to a treatment regimen among adolescents is related to the perceived benefits of compliance.
   *b. adherence to a treatment regimen among adults is related to the perceived benefits of compliance.
   c. adherence to a treatment regimen among adults is related to the perceived costs of compliance.
   d. adolescents who perceive their illness as severe show better adherence to treatment than do those who minimize their illness.

   Page: 222   Topic: Health Beliefs and Attributions

54. The main aim of treatments that help people cope with chronic illness is to
    a. help them find a way to cure their illness.
    b. help them understand their illness.
    *c. reduce stress.
    d. get them to focus on other aspects of their lives.

    Page: 222   Topic: Helping People Cope

55. Friedman and Ulmer's (1984) research with middle-aged heart attack survivors found that
    a. support and attention from the patients' cardiologists reduced the patients' likelihood of having a second heart attack.
    b. monitoring of patients' exercise, medication, and diet reduced their likelihood of having a second heart attack.
    c. advice from cardiologists about exercise, medication, and diet reduced the patients' likelihood of having a second heart attack.
    *d. advice from cardiologists about exercise, medication, and diet combined with continuing counseling on how to relax reduced the patients' likelihood of having a second heart attack.

    Page: 223   Topic: Stress Reduction Through Relaxation

56. People with asthma have been proved to benefit from learning to recognize when their respiratory pathways are narrowing. When they are able to anticipate that their breathing is about to become labored, they can take the appropriate medication to avoid an asthmatic episode. The stress-reduction technique people with asthma use to gain this information is
    *a. biofeedback.
    b. meditation.
    c. progressive relaxation.
    d. cognitive appraisal.

    Page: 224   Topic: Biofeedback

57. Behavioral and cognitive therapy are used to teach people all of the following EXCEPT
    a. stress reduction.
    *b. coming closer to their ideal self.
    c. inculcating new coping skills.
    d. modifying beliefs, cognitions, and emotions.

    Pages: 225–226   Topic: Behavioral and Cognitive-Behavioral Treatment

58. The text suggests that behavioral and cognitive interventions concerning the prevention of HIV infection need to be aimed at all of the following EXCEPT
    a. teaching people the real risks.
    b. modifying health beliefs.
    *c. inducing sufficient fear so that people will use safer-sex practices.
    d. assertiveness training so that people will have the ability to insist on safer-sex practices.

    Pages: 226–227   Topic: Environmental and Community Interventions

59. The coordinated community approach to HIV prevention in San Francisco distributed educational materials aimed at all of the following EXCEPT
    a. warning of the dangers of unprotected sex.
    b. providing instructions on safer sex.
    c. providing instructions on how to use needles.
    *d. warning the community to be careful in their interactions with infected people.

    Page: 227   Topic: Environmental and Community Interventions

60. As aids for coping with stress, the text suggests all of the following EXCEPT
    *a. sticking with the course of action you choose.
    b. appraising the situation and considering alternative actions.
    c. being aware of your defenses.
    d. reducing stress and practicing coping skills.

    Page: 227   Topic: Highlight 5.3: Self-Help in Coping with Stress

TRUE-FALSE QUESTIONS

61. With today's modern technology, it is easier than in years past to distinguish between pure physical illnesses and those with psychological components. (F)

    Page: 195   Topic: Psychosomatic Versus Physical Illness: A Dubious Distinction

62. There is a complex interaction between psychological factors and health. (T)

    Page: 195   Topic: Psychosomatic Versus Physical Illness: A Dubious Distinction

63. According to Freud, conversion hysteria results from childhood emotional traumas. (T)

    Page: 198   Topic: Psychoanalytic Views on the Physical Symptoms of Hysteria

64. Theorists working in the field of psychosomatic medicine have largely abandoned nonspecific stress theory in favor of specificity theory. (F)

    Page: 201   Topic: Specificity Theory

65. Current research has found that Type A personalities are more likely than Type B personalities to suffer from coronary heart disease. (F)

    Pages: 202–203   Topic: Critical Thinking About . . . 5.1: The Rise and Fall (and Rise) of the Type A Behavior Pattern

66. During the resistance stage of the general adaptation syndrome (GAS), there is some cost to the organism for being able to withstand a stressor. (T)

    Page: 201   Topic: Nonspecific Stress Theory

67. Selye agreed with Dunbar and Alexander that the effects of stress are specific. (F)

    Page: 204   Topic: Nonspecific Stress Theory

68. Common life events can make a person ill. (T)

    Page: 206   Topic: Important Life Events

69. People generally can agree on what constitutes a minor violation of the law. (F)

    Page: 210   Topic: Critical Thinking About . . . 5.2: Interpreting Life-Stress Research

70. The inflammation that causes so much pain to arthritis sufferers is exacerbated by daily hassles. (T)

    Page: 209   Topic: Everyday Hassles

71. Tension headaches result from tense muscles in the neck and head, whereas migraine headaches are caused by the contraction and dilation of blood vessels in the head. (F)

    Pages: 211–212   Topic: Chronic Pain and Headaches

72. Vaccinations confer immunity by provoking the formation of memory lymphocytes under controlled conditions. (T)

Page: 213   Topic: Stress and the Immune System

73. Rapid development of the field of psychoneuroimmunology came after Ader and Cohen's (1975) seminal study of suppressing the immune systems of those with schizophrenia. (F)

Page: 213   Topic: Stress and the Immune System

74. Psychoneuroimmunologists have found no relationship between stress and immune functioning among HIV-positive men. (T)

Page: 214   Topic: Stress, Immune Response, and HIV

75. Moderate amounts of stress can help us focus our attention on essential information. (T)

Page: 214   Topic: Effects of Stress on Cognition

76. Clinical studies have found that coping is a more important determinant of blood sugar control among those with diabetes than life-stress is. (F)

Page: 216   Topic: Factors That Modify the Effects of Stress

77. Using denial as a form of coping can be a useful strategy. (T)

Page: 217   Topic: Appraisals

78. Problem-focused coping is a better way to deal with life's problems than is emotion-focused coping. (F)

Page: 217   Topic: Appraisals

79. Toward the end of the baseball season, home teams actually perform better without the social support provided by their hometown crowds. (T)

Page: 219   Topic: Highlight 5.1: When Social Support Increases Stress

80. People who exercise live longer and spend fewer days in hospitals than do those who do not. (T)

Page: 224   Topic: Biofeedback

SHORT-ANSWER QUESTIONS

81. What are the four goals of behavioral medicine?

To learn how psychological factors: (1) make people susceptible (or resistant) to illness, (2) alter the course of an illness, (3) determine compliance with medical treatment, and (4) affect health-related behavior.

Page: 195   Topic: Psychosomatic Versus Physical Illness: A Dubious Distinction

82. List the five disciplines that contribute to behavioral medicine.

psychological and behavioral sciences; social sciences (anthropology, sociology); professional studies (nursing, physical therapy); medical sciences (pathology, radiology); biological sciences (biochemistry, immunology)

Page: 195   Topic: Psychosomatic Versus Physical Illness: A Dubious Distinction

83. Describe the course of Cannon's emergency reaction.

   In the seconds following the perception of a threat, respiration deepens to take in the extra oxygen the muscles need for intense physical effort; an increase in the rate and strength of the heartbeat allows more oxygen to circulate around the body; the spleen contracts and releases oxygen-carrying red blood cells into the bloodstream; the liver releases energy-producing sugar; blood flow to the brain increases; pupils dilate to increase visual acuity; and blood becomes more likely to coagulate, to stop wounds from bleeding.

   Page: 199   Topic: Psychosomatic Medicine

84. What are the two major problems with specificity theory?

   First, researchers did not know what the patients were like before they became ill—having a disease may cause people to act in a particular way, rather than the personality being the causal factor for the disease. Second, the theory assumes that different emotional conflicts have different physiological effects; however, emotions are largely nonspecific and have similar autonomic effects, so it is not normally possible to match specific emotional states with specific disease. It seems more likely that the autonomic arousal produced by emotional turmoil exacerbates a disease.

   Page: 201   Topic: Specificity Theory

85. Explain how hostility, anger, and cynicism make the Type A person more prone to coronary heart disease than the Type B person.

   Hostile, angry people may be more "reactive" to stress; and when they are frustrated or angry, their blood pressure and heart rate increase faster and take longer to return to normal than the Type B person's.

   Page: 203   Topic: Critical Thinking About . . . 5.1: The Rise and Fall (and Rise) of the Type A Behavior Pattern

86. Describe the three stages of Selye's (1950) general adaptation syndrome (GAS).

   Emergency (alarm) reaction: the organism marshals resources to resist the stressor. Resistance stage: the organism uses its physiological resources to minimize tissue damage; neurotransmitters carry mobilization commands to organs around the body; the adrenal gland releases corticosteroids, which further increase blood sugar for energy and reduce inflammation and pain; body functions not directly related to avoiding harm gradually shut down. Exhaustion stage: depletion of body and its defenses; can result in illness or death.

   Pages: 201–202   Topic: Nonspecific Stress Theory

87. Explain the two ways in which psychological variables moderate pain.

   through inhibition of pain impulses; by the production of chemicals called endogenous opioids

   Page: 212   Topic: Chronic Pain and Headaches

88. Explain how the energy response necessary for dealing with stress differs between those with and those without diabetes.

   To mobilize the body's defenses, the GAS requires considerable energy. To obtain this energy, blood sugar levels are increased. Once the stressor is removed, blood sugar levels return to normal in those without diabetes; they remain high, however, in those with diabetes because there is insufficient insulin to reduce them. The resulting excess of blood sugar produces fatigue, irritability, and dehydration and, in severe cases, may cause loss of consciousness or death.

   Page: 212   Topic: Direct Physiological Effects of Stress

89. What are the functions of T cells and B cells in defending against disease?

T cells directly attack foreign invaders, such as bacteria, that make it past the body's first line of defense (the skin and mucous membranes). Foreign substances (antigens) may also provoke B cells to mount an indirect defense by secreting antibodies that bind with the invaders and mark them for later destruction.

Page: 213   Topic: Stress and the Immune System

90. What three components would ideally be included in psychoneuroimmunological research studies? What is the current reality of how these components are included in the research?

The three components are stress, measures of immune system functioning, and measures of health. In practice, most studies have concentrated on the effects of stress on immune functioning or *on the effects of stress on health; studies showing that stress affects healthy people by compromising the immune system are rare.*

Page: 214   Topic: Stress, Immune Response, and HIV

91. Considering the relationship between stress and illness, differentiate successful coping from unsuccessful coping.

Successful coping is marked by compliance with the treatment regimen, by acceptance of the limitations and challenges of the illness, and by attempting to lead as "normal" a life as possible. Unsuccessful coping is evidenced by poor treatment compliance, shame, and social isolation.

Page: 216   Topic: Factors That Modify the Effects of Stress

92. Explain how denial and minimization can be both useful and harmful in terms of dealing with a chronic illness.

If an illness is untreatable, denying the facts may help the ill person make the most of what life remains; but if the condition could be helped by a change in behavior, denial may make matters worse because the person continues to engage in behaviors that exacerbate the illness. Minimizing the seriousness of an illness by seeing it as a minor annoyance may let the person lead a fuller life than would otherwise be the case; but, if carried too far, it can lead people to ignore the limitations imposed by their illness and to take unwise health risks.

Page: 217   Topic: Appraisals

93. Describe the three ways discussed in the text through which social support contributes to health.

First, by providing acceptance, social ties may help maintain self-esteem. Second, friends provide help in times of trouble and sympathetic ears for the expression of painful feelings. Third, members of self-help groups are important sources of new information about disease and its control.

Page: 218   Topic: Social Support

94. Discuss the four issues the text states must be resolved to determine whether a relationship exists among personality, stress, and cancer.

(1) Standard definitions and a standard set of acceptable measures are needed to overcome the problem of inconsistent results. (2) Cancer is a diverse set of conditions. Some may be linked to stress; others may not. By treating different forms of cancer the same, researchers may obscure the true underlying relationships. (3) Cancer develops slowly, and even with the best of prospective studies, it is difficult to make causal links across long periods of time. (4) Although clear links can be seen between certain behaviors and cancer [e.g., the tar in cigarettes], at the present time, there are no definitive human data linking stress, immune suppression, and cancer.

Pages: 220–221   Topic: Highlight 5.2: Personality, Stress, and Cancer

95. What are the six suggestions made in the text for helping yourself cope with stress?

Appraise the situation. Examine your appraisal. Be aware of your defenses. Reduce stress and practice coping skills. Take the necessary actions but do not act impulsively. Remain flexible.

Page: 227   Topic: Highlight 5.3: Self-Help in Coping with Stress

ESSAY QUESTIONS

96. Your roommate has invited you home for dinner. When you get there, you find your friend's mother in a highly anxious state, saying, "I just don't know what everyone expects of me. I work all day, come home to a dirty house, and then I'm expected to make dinner for everyone, and no one helps me out. I just don't know what to do. I am totally stressed out." Then she looks at you and says, "I hear you're a psychology major. Tell me why I'm so stressed out all the time! And, by the way, what in the world *is* stress?" What could you tell her about what stress is and where it comes from?

Discuss the origins, definitions, and theories of stress and the various sources, such as cultural conflict, catastrophes, and daily hassles.

97. In a phone conversation one evening with your mother, she tells you that your cousin's wife has been hospitalized for a stress-related illness, and that the same cousin's sister-in-law jumped out a second-story window because she was "so stressed out." Your mother is sure to tell you (again) that the sister-in-law's mother was an abusive alcoholic while her children were growing up, although she hasn't had a drink for the past 5 years. Knowing that you are studying abnormal psychology, your mother says, "I really don't understand how stress affects physical and psychological health! Will you please explain it to me?"

Explain the direct physiological effects of stress, the relationship between stress and the immune system, and the indirect effects of stress on physical and mental health.

98. As you come into the cafeteria, you notice a couple of your friends in a heated debate. One seems to think that given enough stress, anyone can "crack up." The other says, no, some people are strong enough to withstand anything. The two then get into an argument about early childhood experiences and turn to you to explain why some people end up being mass murderers and others, with similar amounts and kinds of stress in their backgrounds, end up being famous writers or Supreme Court justices. Explain why some people are more prone to suffer from the effects of stress than others.

Discuss the various factors that modify the effects of stress, such as appraisals, social support, and individual characteristics.

99. Your high school counselor hears that you are now a psychology major and that you are taking this class in abnormal psychology. She calls you and asks you to talk to the students at your old high school about what steps they can take to deal with their stress. What would you tell these students?

First, explain the sources of stress and Lazarus's work on coping styles. Then provide approaches that help people cope, such as relaxation, behavioral and cognitive-behavioral treatments, social support, and the six suggestions given for self-help in coping with stress.

100. An old friend of yours from high school calls to tell you that someone in your class has cancer. Your friend says to you, "Well, you know, she always had the kind of personality that's linked with getting cancer." What could you tell your friend about the link between personality traits and cancer?

Discuss the research on personality, stress, and chronic illness and the problems with finding direct links between stress, the immune system, and chronic illness.

CHAPTER 6
THE SUBSTANCE DISORDER SPECTRUM

MULTIPLE-CHOICE QUESTIONS

1. The largest single category of psychological disorders is _____ disorders.
   *a. substance-related
   b. schizophrenic
   c. mood
   d. anxiety

   Page: 232   Topic: Introduction

2. Alexandra's science teacher told her class that most of them consume psychoactive substances daily, even though they are legal. This would include all of the following EXCEPT
   a. coffee.
   *b. lemonade.
   c. cocoa.
   d. chocolate.

   Page: 233   Topic: The Substance Spectrum: Most Common Psychoactive Substances Used by American College Students

3. Bruce confided in a friend that he was using MDMA, saying it was "really cool." His friend, who had researched the effects of psychoactive drugs in a science class, told Bruce this was an unhealthy thing to do to his body and his mind because MDMA is
   a. an opioid.
   b. an amphetamine.
   *c. a hallucinogen.
   d. a sedative.

   Page: 233   Topic: The Substance Spectrum: Most Common Psychoactive Substances Used by American College Students

4. Breathable chemical vapors produced by substances such as paint thinners, dry-cleaning fluid, and gasoline are called
   a phencyclidines.
   b. anxiolytics.
   c. hallucinogens.
   *d. inhalants.

   Pages: 232–233   Topic: Agony of a Gasoline Sniffer

5. Six-year-old Joaquin lives on the streets. He inhales glue and paint and suffers from substance intoxication. The symptoms we would see in Joaquin are
   *a. mood lability, belligerence, cognitive impairment, and impaired social functioning.
   b. malnutrition, lack of hygiene, and impaired social functioning.
   c. delusions, hallucinations, skin rashes, and cognitive impairment.
   d. negativity, malnutrition, drowsiness, and nausea.

   Page: 233   Topic: Agony of a Gasoline Sniffer

6. In the case study of Davey Blackthunder, it was clear from the interview between the social worker and Davey's father and uncle that a critical underlying issue to be dealt with (besides Davey's substance disorder) was
    a. the family structure.
    *b. cultural sensitivity.
    c. Davey's education.
    d. unemployment.

    Pages: 234–235   Topic: Document 6.2: Excerpt from Social Work Conference . . .

7. A persistent symptom that Davey Blackthunder had experienced over the years he had been sniffing gasoline was
    a. believing he was God.
    b. hearing voices.
    *c. seeing ghosts.
    d. delirium.

    Pages: 234–235   Topic: Document 6.2: Excerpts from Social Work Conference . . .

8. The text states that the main reasons for using any substance include all of the following EXCEPT
    a. altering one's psychological state.
    b. achieving peer group acceptance.
    c. sharing a social activity.
    *d. rebelling against societal values.

    Page: 237   Topic: Psychoactive Substances Are Ubiquitous

9. The substances most frequently used by American college students are
    *a. caffeine, alcohol, nicotine, and marijuana.
    b. alcohol, marijuana, and cocaine.
    c. caffeine, alcohol, and heroin.
    d. nicotine, alcohol, and cocaine.

    Page: 237   Topic: Psychoactive Substances Are Ubiquitous

10. The first people to drink caffeine were the
    a. Incas.
    *b. Chinese.
    c. Russians.
    d. Arabs.

    Page: 237   Topic: Caffeine

11. The world's most popular source of caffeine today is
    a. chocolate.
    b. tea.
    *c. coffee.
    d. cola drinks.

    Page: 238   Topic: Caffeine

12. Chemicals that reduce the potency of other chemicals are referred to as
    a. stimulants.
    b. protagonists.
    c. diuretics
    *d. antagonists.

    Page: 239   Topic: Caffeine/Action

13. Using caffeine in sports
    *a. can be dangerous because the physical exertion of sports causes intense sweating, and caffeine increases the excretion of liquid from the body, which can result in severe dehydration.
    b. can be extremely helpful because the stimulating action of caffeine enhances the athlete's ability to perform.
    c. has been shown to have little effect because caffeine is such a mild substance that it neither adds to nor detracts from an athlete's ability to perform.
    d. produces an energy spurt 45 to 60 minutes after it is taken, so its effect is difficult to ascertain.

    Page: 239   Topic: Caffeine/Action

14. Caffeine works as a stimulant in part by
    a. diminishing the inhibitory effect of neurotransmitters that calm people down, such as serotonin.
    *b. increasing the activity of glutamate, norepinephrine, and serotonin, which combine to make people more aroused.
    c. reducing breathing problems, thereby pumping more oxygen-rich blood through the system.
    d. increasing the flow of blood to the central and autonomic nervous systems, thus energizing the body and brain.

    Page: 239   Topic: Caffeine/Action

15. Amphetamines were originally intended as a medication to treat
    a. attention deficit disorder.
    b. narcolepsy.
    *c. asthma.
    d. obesity.

    Page: 239   Topic: Table 6.3: Examples of Stimulants . . .

16. Teresa began taking amphetamines to help her lose weight. She found that they made her feel alert, energized, strong, and happy, and she believes she is able to study better and longer. Unfortunately, she may experience many dangerous side effects that include all of the following EXCEPT
    a. malnutrition and dehydration.
    b. severe anxiety and cognitive distortions such as hallucinations.
    c. death.
    *d. stomach cancer.

    Page: 239   Topic: Table 6.3: Examples of Stimulants . . .

17. Doreen has started to use cocaine. Continued use may have which of the following direct effects on her health?
    *a. a psychotic disorder
    b. obsessive-compulsive behavior
    c. hepatitis
    d. catatonia

    Page: 239   Topic: Table 6.3: Examples of Stimulants . . . /Cocaine

18. A stimulant that was once used in a popular soft drink is
    a. amphetamines.
    *b. cocaine.
    c. nicotine.
    d. cocoa.

    Page: 239   Topic: Table 6.3: Examples of Stimulants . . . /Cocaine

19. Anabolic steroids, the modern version of ancient potions taken to ensure victory in sporting events or battle, made their first appearance in the 1950s with which Olympic team?
    a. Japanese sumo wrestlers
    b. American javelin throwers
    *c. Russian weight lifters
    d. Canadian hockey players

    Page: 240   Topic: Highlight 6.1: Threatening Mind and Body

20. Anabolic steroids work as agents to increase size and strength by
    a. processing fat into muscle.
    b. retaining carbohydrates, which accelerates the growth of muscles and tendons.
    c. improving appetite and metabolic functioning.
    *d. retaining protein, which accelerates the growth of muscles, bones, and skin.

    Page: 240   Topic: Highlight 6.1: Threatening Mind and Body

21. Arnold has been taking anabolic steroids for more than a year. He can expect all of the following side effects EXCEPT
    *a. increased urination.
    b. impotence.
    c. sudden rages of anger.
    d. liver damage.

    Page: 240   Topic: Highlight 6.1: Threatening Mind and Body

22. Winston uses a substance that provides as much income for governments, by way of taxation, as it does for the people who produce and sell it. This substance is
    a. alcohol.
    *b. nicotine.
    c. cocaine.
    d. morphine.

    Page: 241   Topic: Nicotine

23. What is the relationship between most forms of substance use and income and level of education?
    a. Substance use increases as income increases but decreases as level of education rises.
    b. Substance use increases as income and level of education increase.
    *c. Substance use decreases as income and level of education increase.
    d. There is no relationship between substance use and income and level of education.

    Page: 241   Topic: Nicotine

24. Which of the following substances contained in cigarettes have NOT been shown to be present at levels high enough to be definitely linked to disease?
    a. tar
    b. carbon monoxide
    c. formaldehyde
    *d. nicotine

    Page: 242   Topic: Nicotine/Health Effects

25. With respect to the link between smoking and cancer, Hans Eysenck argued that
    *a. cancer occurs most often in people with genetically determined cancer-prone personalities.
    b. cigarette smoking is a direct cause of lung cancer, as well as cancer of the mouth, throat, and larynx.
    c. whether a smoker develops cancer depends on where they stand on other factors, such as pollution and diet.
    d. whether a smoker develops cancer depends primarily on hereditary factors.

    Page: 243   Topic: Nicotine/Health Effects

26. Although caffeine and nicotine are stimulants, they are perceived to be calming. What is the physiological explanation for this paradox?
    a. In addition to their stimulant properties, caffeine and nicotine also contain chemical properties that calm the individual.
    *b. Caffeine and nicotine stimulate the release of the body's natural opioids, thereby reducing anxiety.
    c. The explanation involves the rebound effect: After the initial stimulation of the sympathetic nervous system, the parasympathetic nervous system engages to calm the person.
    d. There is no physiological effect; the calming is a psychological effect that results from expectancies and social reinforcement.

    Page: 244   Topic: Nicotine/Health Effects

27. Sandra, a sophomore in college, has recently learned in her psychology and health science classes that NIDA surveys (1994, 1996) found that more than _____% of college students reported using alcohol in the past month.
    a. 95
    b. 80
    *c. 65
    d. 50

    Page: 244   Topic: Alcohol

28. Who of the following is most likely to be a heavy drinker?
    a. Pamela, a 54-year-old White female with a master's degree in economics.
    b. Arnold, a 70-year-old White male retired postal worker who did not go to college.
    c. John, a 26-year-old African American male who started his restaurant business after graduating from high school.
    *d. Alexander, a 20-year-old White male college student.

    Page: 244   Topic: Alcohol

29. The prohibition against alcohol in the United States from 1920 to 1933 was prompted by
    *a. a war against sin.
    b. the Industrial Revolution.
    c. high increases in alcohol-related deaths.
    d. economics.

    Page: 245   Topic: Alcohol

30. Adrienne has used a substance that lowers her arousal and makes her drowsy. It also results in the loss of some degree of self-control. The substance Adrienne used is most likely
    a. nicotine.
    *b. alcohol.
    c. cocaine.
    d. amphetamines.

    Page: 245   Topic: Alcohol/Action

31. All of the following effects have been found for sedatives and anxiolytics EXCEPT:
    a. mixing them with alcohol is potentially lethal.
    b. they depress bodily functions.
    *c. their use results in depression.
    d. abrupt cessation of these drugs after prolonged use can cause seizures.

    Page: 246   Topic: Table 6.5: Depressants Other Than Alcohol

32. Dwayne, a chronic user of heroin, can expect to have a shorter life expectancy than his age peers who do not use opioids for all of the following reasons EXCEPT:
    a. he may overdose.
    b. by sharing needles with other users, he may contract HIV.
    c. as a heroin user, he is likely to live in a dangerous world and is thus more likely than nonusers to be the victim of a homicide.
    *d. the drug used to reverse an overdose (Narcan) can have harmful and even fatal side effects.

    Page: 246   Topic: Table 6.5: Depressants Other Than Alcohol

33. Jimmy was a heavy drinker from the time he was in junior high school. After years of drinking, he developed liver disease, hepatitis, and severe malnutrition. Toward the end of his life, he also became confused and disoriented, developed double vision, and suffered memory loss due to a largely irreversible type of dementia referred to as
    *a. Wernicke-Korsakoff syndrome.
    b. AIDS.
    c. cirrhosis.
    d. Alzheimer's disease.

    Page: 246   Topic: Alcohol/Health Effects

34. Because his mother was a heavy drinker who consumed alcohol during her pregnancy, Adam was born with facial deformities, heart defects, and organ malfunctions. He was also retarded and hyperactive. This totally preventable disease is called
    a. Down syndrome.
    *b. fetal alcohol syndrome.
    c. Klinefelter's syndrome.
    d. Wernicke-Korsakoff syndrome.

    Page: 247   Topic: Alcohol/Health Effects

35. The concentration of alcohol in the blood can be expected to affect judgment and motor coordination when it reaches a level of _____% of the blood by volume.
    a. .01
    *b. .05
    c. .10
    d. .15

    Page: 247   Topic: Alcohol/Psychological Effects

36. What trend has been seen for cannabis use among young people in the past few decades?
    a. Its use has declined steadily since the 1960s.
    b. Its use has increased steadily since the 1960s.
    *c. From 1979 to 1992, its use declined, but its use has increased through the 1990s.
    d. From 1979 to 1992, its use increased, but its use has decreased through the 1990s.

    Page: 248   Topic: Cannabis

37. Although cannabis can produce hallucinations, it is not categorized as a hallucinogen in the *DSM-IV* because
    a. there is a strong group of activists who are lobbying to decriminalize its use, and they want to keep it separate from other hallucinogens.
    b. it has been found to alleviate symptoms of certain illnesses and side effects of certain medications.
    c. the hallucinations it produces are significantly different from the types of hallucinations seen with the hallucinogens.
    *d. perceptual distortions do not always accompany cannabis intoxication.

    Page: 248   Topic: Cannabis

38. John, a musician and writer, says that hallucinogens help his creative process. His hallucinogen of preference, a cactus derivative, is called:
    *a. mescaline.
    b. psilocybin.
    c. MDMA.
    d. LSD.

    Page: 249   Topic: Table 6.6: Common Hallucinogenic Substances

39. Angel used a drug that was developed as a surgical anesthetic in the 1950s. Although he took the drug to experience hallucinations, on several occasions it caused him to go into a psychotic state, impairing his judgment so extensively that he ultimately committed suicide. This drug is
    a. lysergic acid diethylamide.
    *b. phencyclidine.
    c. mescaline.
    d. psilocybin.

    Page: 249   Topic: Table 6.6: Common Hallucinogenic Substances

40. The ban on cannabis during the first half of the 20th century was largely uncontroversial because
    a. few people were aware of its medicinal properties.
    b. the people who were using it could afford the fine if they were caught.
    *c. it was used primarily by a rural ethnic minority.
    d. it was used primarily by bohemians, who were seen as outsiders and deviants.

    Page: 250   Topic: Cannabis

41. Within a few minutes of inhaling cannabis smoke
    a. users experience decreased heartbeat.
    b. users experience decreased blood pressure.
    c. blood vessels in the eye contract.
    *d. THC binds to nerve cell receptors.

    Page: 250   Topic: Cannabis/Action

42. In the 18th century, doctors prescribed cannabis for
    *a. coughs, venereal disease, and headaches.
    b. healing peptic ulcers and increasing sex drive.
    c. treating asthma and other respiratory diseases.
    d. improving creativity.

    Page: 252   Topic: Highlight 6.2: Substances, Medicine, and Morality

43. Research has found all of the following health benefits for cannabis use EXCEPT
    a. suppressing the nausea caused by anti-cancer and anti-AIDS treatments.
    *b. treating venereal diseases such as gonorrhea and herpes.
    c. preventing damage to optic nerves by reducing excess pressure in the eyeballs of patients with glaucoma.
    d. reducing the pain suffered by people with multiple sclerosis.

    Page: 253   Topic: Highlight 6.2: Substances, Medicine, and Morality

44. Whereas many psychoactive substances induce paranoia in their users, the text notes that cannabis has the same effect on
    a. medical practitioners.
    b. insurance carriers.
    *c. governments.
    d. people using it medicinally.

    Page: 253   Topic: Highlight 6.2: Substances, Medicine, and Morality

45. Before people will use a substance, they must first
    a. be able to afford it.
    b. have a physiological need for it.
    c. develop expectancies about what it will do.
    *d. know that the substance exists and have access to it.

    Page: 251   Topic: Modeling and Availability

46. Exposure to which substance typically comes later than exposure to the others?
    *a. cannabis
    b. nicotine
    c. caffeine
    d. alcohol

    Page: 252   Topic: Modeling and Availability

47. Colleen, a college junior, is LEAST likely to use which substance?
    a. caffeine
    *b. amphetamines
    c. alcohol
    d. nicotine

    Page: 254   Topic: Modeling and Availability

48. A critical factor that determines whether we continue to use substances once we start is
    a. increased cognitive abilities.
    b. lack of monitoring by our parents.
    *c. stimulation of the brain's pleasure center.
    d. how easy it is to get the substance.

    Page: 254   Topic: Reinforcement

49. Davey Blackthunder was encouraged by his friends to inhale gasoline. At first, they said things like this to him: "Come on and try it. Are you chicken?" Davey's yielding to this type of social pressure demonstrates
    a. modeling.
    b. expectancies.
    c. positive reinforcement.
    *d. negative reinforcement.

    Page: 255   Topic: Reinforcement

50. A historical reason for the high use of substances among Native American populations is that
   *a. Europeans sometimes used substances as a way of subduing indigenous peoples.
   b. indigenous peoples have had a history of poverty and poor employment prospects.
   c. having developed a sense of despair after being colonized, indigenous peoples look for a way out.
   d. Western-style interventions are not typically appropriate to tribal cultures.

   Page: 256   Topic: Social and Cultural Context

51. Evidence for a predisposition to substances has been found in:
   a. research with female twins.
   *b. research with male twins.
   c. studies of first-degree relatives.
   d. studies of family histories.

   Page: 256   Topic: Biological Variables and Individual Differences

52. According to Blum and his colleagues (1996), the DRD2 gene
   a. indicates which individuals are going to become alcoholics.
   b. indicates which individuals are going to have problems with substance abuse.
   *c. could mark a "reward deficiency syndrome."
   d. is one of several genes that have been implicated in substance abuse.

   Page: 256   Topic: Biological Variables and Individual Differences

53. John, who is of average height and weight, amazes all of his friends by being able to drink all evening and never appear to get drunk. John has apparently developed
   a. dependence on alcohol.
   b. an immunity to alcohol.
   c. an opponent-process reaction to alcohol.
   *d. a tolerance to alcohol.

   Page: 257   Topic: Potential Problems of Sustained Substance Use

54. After smoking two packs of cigarettes a day for 17 years, Anita decided to quit smoking. She chose not to use a nicotine patch or any specific program, but just to stop and not ever have another cigarette. Her friends have noticed that Anita has become irritable, restless, and distractible, and she is always hungry. It appears that Anita is going through
   *a. nicotine withdrawal syndrome.
   b. "cold turkey" syndrome.
   c. the opponent-process reaction.
   d. tolerance.

   Page: 258   Topic: Potential Problems of Sustained Substance Use

55. The positive effects produced by psychoactive substances are often followed by negative feelings—or "highs" are often followed by "crashes." According to _____, this is a natural aspect of self-regulation.
   a. tolerance theory
   *b. opponent-process theory
   c. withdrawal theory
   d. the general adaptation syndrome

   Page: 258   Topic: Potential Problems of Sustained Substance Use

56. As stated in the text, according to the *DSM-IV* diagnostic criteria for substance abuse, all of the following substances may be abused EXCEPT

    a.   alcohol.

    b.   gasoline.

  *c.   caffeine

    d.   marijuana.

Page: 258   Topic: Substance Use Versus Substance Abuse

57. Timothy has been using LSD for 20 years on a regular basis. He has begun to organize his life around satisfying his craving. His friends believe he is addicted. The *DSM-IV* term for this would be substance

    a.   use.

    b.   abuse.

    c.   tolerance.

  *d.   dependence.

Page: 260   Topic: Substance Dependence

58. Frank realized that he had become addicted to caffeine. He drank several caffeinated soft drinks each day to help him stay awake and alert, and he became irritable and began to shake if he ran out of these beverages. Finally, he decided that it was time to think about changing his habits and switching to water instead, so he began to make a plan to do that in the next couple of months. Which of Lichtenstein and Glasgow's (1992) stages is Frank in?

  *a.   contemplation

    b.   precontemplation

    c.   action

    d.   maintenance

Page: 261   Topic: Stages in Overcoming Substance Dependence

59. Chance decided, after 20 years on heroin, that it was time to give it up. Although his doctor urged him to go into a residential program, he decided to ask his mother if he could quit at her home and if she would take care of him during the process. She agreed and nursed him through. This painful period during which Chance stopped taking heroin and the drug was removed from his body is called

    a.   rehabilitation.

  *b.   detoxification.

    c.   cleansing.

    d.   antagonism.

Page: 261   Topic: Detoxification

60. A drug that is used to block the action of opioids, to assist people who are dependent on alcohol, and to assist in the treatment of substance abuse is

    a.   Antabuse.

    b.   ipecac.

  *c.   naltrexone.

    d.   methadone.

Page: 262   Topic: Antagonist and Aversive Drugs

61. Antoinette was not able to attend her drug rehabilitation program every day because of her work and family obligations. Instead, she arranged with the program to come in three times a week for her medication. As a heroin user, it is most likely that she was being treated with
    a. Antabuse.
    b. naltrexone.
    c. methadone.
    *d. LAAM.

    Page: 262   Topic: Substance Replacement and Maintenance

62. Davey Blackthunder received many different types of treatment for his dependence on gasoline sniffing and other substances, each aimed at addressing another reason for his dependence. This is referred to as _____ treatment.
    *a. multimodal
    b. eclectic
    c. multimethod
    d. intermodal

    Page: 263   Topic: Multimodal Treatment

63. One important reason so many therapists favor the multimodal approach to treatment is that
    a. they typically take a team perspective and strive to satisfy the preferences of all the team members.
    *b. there is a lack of evidence favoring one treatment approach over another, so therapists use several to be sure something will work.
    c. the research suggests that using several different types of therapy is superior to using only one approach.
    d. it is only in this way that they can be sure to include both therapy and cultural sensitivity.

    Page: 264   Topic: Multimodal Treatment

64. Dale is in therapy for his dependence on marijuana, which is interfering with his studies, his work, and his family life. The therapist teaches Dale self-statements that stress the negative health consequences of substance dependence and the benefits of quitting. She also uses role playing to teach Dale how to reject the marijuana his friends offer him, and she has Dale sign a contract giving his approval for her to notify his employer if he backslides. The type of therapy Dale is receiving is
    a. psychoanalytic.
    b. humanistic.
    *c. cognitive-behavioral.
    d. behavioral.

    Pages: 263–264   Topic: Document 6.6: Alan Arnold's Treatment Plan for Davey Blackthunder

65. Dr. Janes is designing a study of treatment effectiveness. To evaluate treatment effectiveness, she will need to consider all of the following issues EXCEPT
    a. a definition of the treatment population.
    b. procedures for people who drop out of the study.
    c. a definition of success.
    *d. demographic differences among participants.

    Page: 264   Topic: Critical Thinking About . . . 6.1: Assessing Treatment Outcome

66. Who is most likely to be a mentally ill chemical abuser?
    *a. Glen, a 25-year-old male who is homeless, has hepatitis, and was arrested for burglary
    b. Vera, a 25-year-old female who is homeless, has tuberculosis, and was arrested for shoplifting
    c. Avery, a 65-year-old male who is poor and has a history of childhood illnesses
    d. Gwen, a 55-year old single female who lives with her daughter and granddaughter

    Page: 266   Topic: Treatment of Substance Dependence: State of the Art

67. With respect to the legal approaches to primary prevention of substance abuse,
    a. the most effective approach has been prohibition.
    *b. legalization of psychoactive substances has not been viewed favorably in the United States.
    c. the most effective approach has been restricting access.
    d. most of the approaches have been at least somewhat effective.

    Page: 267   Topic: Legal Restrictions

68. The text gives all of the following reasons that some psychoactive substances are illegal EXCEPT:
    a. they pose a serious danger to individuals or to society.
    b. to keep people from becoming substance dependent and having their lives ruined.
    *c. using psychoactive substances is morally wrong.
    d. dependency has a high social cost.

    Page: 268   Topic: Highlight 6.3: Minimizing Harm

69. The main value of health warnings is to
    a. make people aware of the dangers of psychoactive substances.
    b. frighten people into discontinuing use of psychoactive substances.
    c. present an image of concern so that the public believes that the government is trying to do something about the problem.
    *d. move users from the precontemplative to the contemplative stage of the substance-quitting process.

    Page: 267   Topic: Global Educational Programs

70. A specific educational intervention designed by Goldstein, Reagles, and Amann (1990)
    *a. attempts to teach children and adolescents the skills necessary to refuse substances.
    b. uses aversive techniques to teach children and adolescents to refrain from using substances.
    c. provides extensive information about the social, biological, and psychological consequences of using substances.
    d. brings children and adolescents to mental hospitals, jails, and drug treatment facilities to demonstrate the consequences of using substances.

    Page: 267   Topic: Specific Educational Programs

71. All of the following are integral to effective prevention programs EXCEPT
    a. being long-term and extending over the school career with repeat interventions.
    *b. implementing harsh penalties for substance use.
    c. teaching children and adolescents the skills necessary to refuse substances.
    d. involving parents as well as children and adolescents in the program.

    Pages: 267 and 269   Topic: Specific Educational Programs

72. All of the following are considered minimum-cost interventions EXCEPT
    a. family doctors.
    b. worksite programs.
    *c. treatment facilities.
    d. self-help.

    Pages: 269 and 271   Topic: Minimum-Cost Interventions

TRUE-FALSE QUESTIONS

73. There is no precise boundary between social drinking and alcohol abuse. (T)

    Page: 232   Topic: Introduction

74. As stated in the text, caffeine and heroin have little in common. (F)

    Page: 232   Topic: Introduction

75. More than 90% of adults in North America consume caffeine regularly. (T)

  Page: 237   Topic: Caffeine

76. Coffee belongs to the same class of chemicals as amphetamines. (T)

  Page: 238   Topic: Caffeine/Action

77. Despite the health hazards posed by anabolic steroids, men take them not only to increase their physical strength but also to combat impotence. (F)

  Page: 240   Topic: Highlight 6.1: Threatening Mind and Body

78. Caffeine is used by many people to relax or even to help them sleep. (T)

  Page: 241   Topic: Caffeine/Psychological Effects

79. Overall, tobacco use has decreased for males but has increased for females since the 1960s. (F)

  Page: 241   Topic: Nicotine

80. Nicotine is so toxic that it has been used as a natural insecticide. (T)

  Page: 241   Topic: Nicotine/Action

81. Drinking black coffee is probably the most effective way to sober up after consuming alcohol. (F)

  Page: 245   Topic: Alcohol/Action

82. The reason smaller people reach the .05 level of blood alcohol sooner than larger people is that bigger people have more blood. (T)

  Page: 248   Topic: Alcohol/Psychological Effects

83. The government's reason for refusing to legalize the medical use of cannabis is that the substance has never been shown to have any positive medical benefits. (F)

  Pages: 252–253   Topic: Highlight 6.2: Substances, Medicine, and Morality

84. Substances such as nicotine and caffeine that are used as stimulants can also be used to help people relax. (T)

  Page: 255   Topic: Expectancies

85. Some people may be genetically programmed to favor certain substances. (T)

  Page: 256   Topic: Biological Variables and Individual Differences

86. The existence of the DRD2 gene shows that some people are born alcoholics. (F)

  Page: 256   Topic: Biological Variables and Individual Differences

87. As tolerance to a substance develops, chronic users require less of the substance to produce any effect. (F)

  Page: 257   Topic: Potential Problems of Sustained Substance Use

88. According to the *DSM-IV*, psychological dependence can occur without physiological dependence. (T)

  Page: 258   Topic: Substance Dependence

89. Remedies such as Antabuse for alcoholism and silver nitrate gum for smokers have been effective in helping unmotivated people reduce their dependence. (F)

  Page: 262   Topic: Antagonist and Aversive Drugs

90. Outcome studies have found relapse prevention programs to be highly effective. (F)

    Page: 265   Topic: Relapse Prevention

91. Long-term follow-ups for treatment of heroin dependence show a majority of users are dead, in jail, or still abusing heroin. (T)

    Page: 265   Topic: Treatment of Substance Dependence: State of the Art

92. In the future, it will be necessary to show not only that psychological treatments are effective in reducing substance use, but also that these treatments are cost-effective. (T)

    Page: 270   Topic: Critical Thinking About . . . 6.2: Cost-Effectiveness Analysis

SHORT-ANSWER QUESTIONS

93. State the three main reasons noted in the text for using *any* substance.

    The substance allows the user to alter his or her psychological state (to get "high") while also providing peer group acceptance and, at least initially, a shared social activity.

    Page: 237   Topic: Psychoactive Substances Are Ubiquitous

94. What are the potential health dangers of using anabolic steroids?

    In men, anabolic steroids shrink the testicles and reduce sperm count; they also produce impotence, baldness, and difficulty urinating. Because they are derived from the male sex hormone, they foster masculine characteristics, so women who take them develop facial hair and deeper voices, and their breasts shrink. In both males and females, anabolic steroids produce acne, tremors, high blood pressure, and liver damage; and in children they can halt growth. They also affect mood, causing "roid rage," in which anger erupts suddenly and may lead to violence; withdrawal results in deep depression. Users who share needles to inject steroids increase their exposure to HIV; and black market steroids are often contaminated with poisonous materials.

    Page: 240   Topic: Highlight 6.1: Threatening Mind and Body

95. Explain the two reasons smokers who had contracted cancer were unsuccessful in early lawsuits against the tobacco companies, and the judicial shift that reversed this trend.

    First, it is difficult to prove that any particular person's illness was the result of smoking and not some other factors; and second, people voluntarily chose to smoke even though cigarette packages contained health warnings. In 1992, the U.S. Supreme Court ruled that manufacturers could be held liable if it could be proved that they had deliberately conspired to misrepresent the dangers of smoking.

    Page: 242   Topic: Nicotine/Health Effects

96. Explain the effects of alcohol on a person's body and behavior.

    One of the most important effects that alcohol has on the central nervous system is reducing inhibition (controlled by the GABA neurotransmitter system), resulting in loss of some degree of self-control. The effects of alcohol in the sympathetic nervous system and the body's organ systems are dilation of blood vessels, increased blood pressure, lowered heart rate, and slower respiration. Most of the ingested alcohol goes to the liver, where it is gradually metabolized and excreted.

    Page: 245   Topic: Alcohol/Action

97. Explain why African American women and women members of certain Native American tribes are more likely to have children with fetal alcohol syndrome than are members of other groups. What other factors are important in terms of how a person responds to alcohol?

The increased vulnerability of African American and some Native American women appears to be the result of genetic differences in alcohol metabolism, underscoring that an individual's response to alcohol is not just a function of how much the person drinks, but also genetic endowment, nutritional status, size, diet, and other factors.

Page: 247   Topic: Alcohol/Health Effects

98. What are the five primary factors discussed in the text that explain why people use psychoactive substances?

exposure and availability; reinforcement; expectancies; social and cultural context; biological variables

Page: 251   Topic: Why Are Psychoactive Substances So Popular?

99. Explain how a substance, such as caffeine or nicotine, that stimulates and arouses bodily functions can help people relax and fall asleep?

First, increases in arousal are reinforcing for low-arousal people, and stimulants affect the brain's pleasure center by releasing pleasurable endorphins. Second, cognitive expectancies are such that if we believe that a cup of tea will help us sleep or that a cigarette will help us relax, then they probably will have these effects even though both contain stimulants.

Page: 255   Topic: Expectancies

100. Identify the two different types of people discussed in the text who develop problems with alcohol.

One group has the DRD2 gene and a family history of excessive drinking; they develop alcohol-related problems early in life. The second group does not have the gene, their drinking problems develop late in life, and their social and occupational functioning is only mildly affected. Drinking in the second group seems to be affected mainly by environmental factors (exposure, social reinforcement), whereas drinking in the first group may be influenced more by genetics.

Page: 256   Topic: Biological Variables and Individual Differences

101. What is the opponent-process theory?

The positive effects produced by psychoactive substances are often followed by negative feelings—or "highs" are often followed by "crashes." This shifting between positive and negative feelings is a natural aspect of self-regulation. As tolerance develops, chronic substance users require increasing amounts of a substance to produce any effect. As the effect wears off, the person experiences withdrawal symptoms, including an intense craving for the substance. Eventually, the substance no longer produces any positive feeling of elation, but users continue to use it to satisfy the craving. At this point, the motivation for taking the substance has moved from positive (to get high) to negative (to satisfy a craving/avoid withdrawal symptoms).

Pages: 257–258   Topic: Potential Problems of Sustained Substance Use

102. Describe the characteristics of the substances that are most likely to produce dependence.

They have social reinforcing qualities, such as peer acceptance; they produce tolerance; they produce withdrawal symptoms; they lead to significant mood changes; and they affect pain, alertness, arousal, or stress.

Pages: 258 and 260   Topic: Substance Dependence

103. What happens during each of the four stages in Lichtenstein and Glasgow's (1992) model for giving up a substance?

From not even thinking about giving up (the precontemplation stage), people move through the contemplation stage, in which they are thinking about giving up the substance in the next 6 months, to the action stage (in which they actually quit). In the final, maintenance, stage, they consolidate their treatment gains and attempt to avoid relapse.

Page: 261   Topic: Stages in Overcoming Substance Dependence

104. What is the general idea behind the multimodal treatment approach?

The idea is to wean people away from a substance; help them manage their craving; and give them the skills necessary to cope with social stress, anxiety, and other potential causes of substance abuse.

Page: 263   Topic: Multimodal Treatment

105. Explain the five specific cognitive-behavioral interventions discussed in the text that were used to help Davey Blackthunder abstain from using inhalants.

Cognitive self-statements: teach self-statements that stress the negative health consequences of substance dependence and the benefits of quitting. Social skills: through role playing, teach Davey how to reject substances offered by friends. Relaxation training: teach systematic relaxation to show Davey how to relax without the aid of substances. Behavioral contracting: offer a contract in which he will receive privileges for staying substance free and will sacrifice privileges if he backslides. Aversive conditioning: later in treatment, use rapid smoking to create an aversive reaction to tobacco to help Davey stop smoking.

Pages: 263–264   Topic: Document 6.6: Alan Arnold's Treatment Plan for Davey Blackthunder

106. Discuss the five types of choices researchers must make when designing a study of treatment effectiveness.

First, they must define the treatment population. Then they must decide how to deal with people who drop out of treatment before the end of the program. Third, they must decide on a definition of success. Fourth, they must give their outcome criterion an operational definition and decide how they will collect their data (e.g., self-report, biochemical tests). Finally, they must decide how long to follow-up on their participants.

Pages: 264–265   Topic: Critical Thinking About . . . 6.1: Assessing Treatment Outcome

107. Explain the three reasons the text gives for the illegality of some psychoactive substances.

They pose a serious danger to individuals or to society; to keep people from becoming substance dependent and having their lives ruined; the high social cost of dependency.

Page: 268   Topic: Highlight 6.3: Minimizing Harm

ESSAY QUESTIONS

108. One of your friends from class is a foreign exchange student. She has read the chapter about substance disorders and comes to you somewhat confused. She says that in her country no one would ever consider doing something so harmful as taking psychoactive substances, and she asks you to explain why psychoactive substances are so popular. What could you tell her?

Discuss modeling and availability, reinforcement, expectancies, social and cultural context, and biological variables and individual differences.

109. Your 12-year-old cousin has been suspended from school for smoking marijuana in the boys' bathroom. His mother has asked you to talk to him about the dangers of using drugs. What would you say to him?

Discuss the health effects of common substances as well as their psychological effects, and the potential problems of substance use/abuse/dependence.

110. Having heard that you are taking this class in abnormal psychology, your high school counselor calls to ask that you talk to a group of students who are having problems related to their substance use. He wants you to tell them about the various treatment options that are available to them for overcoming substance dependence. What would you tell them?

Address the stages in overcoming substance dependence, detoxification, antagonist and aversive drugs, substance replacement and maintenance, self-help groups, multimodal treatment, relapse prevention, and the current information concerning how effective treatment is—or is not. Be sure to look at the downside of the various treatments.

111. A local religious group is concerned about the potential for members of their youth groups to become involved in using psychoactive substances. The head of the congregation has asked you for advice on prevention tactics. What would you suggest?

Bring up the various methods of prevention, addressing those that are and are not effective, including legal restrictions (not very effective), global educational programs, specific educational programs, and minimum-cost interventions. Be sure to talk about the importance of including the entire family in the educational programs.

112. As you come into the cafeteria, you see two classmates arguing about treatment effectiveness for substance use disorders. They can't seem to agree on how to assess treatment effectiveness, or whether it's worthwhile even to bother to treat someone with such a disorder. They turn to you for your opinion. What would you tell them?

Go into the various types of treatment, emphasizing the importance of the multimodal approach; then discuss the various issues involved in assessing treatment outcome and the cost-effectiveness analysis.

CHAPTER 7
DISSOCIATIVE, SOMATOFORM,
AND FACTITIOUS DISORDERS

MULTIPLE-CHOICE QUESTIONS

1. In the introductory story about Freud and the young man on the train, the young man indicated his curiosity about why he had omitted a word (*aliquis*) from a quote. The technique Freud used to understand this memory lapse is
    *a. free association.
    b. dream analysis.
    c. interpretation of transference.
    d. hypnosis.

    Page: 276   Topic: Introduction

2. In the introductory story about Freud and the young man on the train, Freud used the example to support his theory that
    a. slips of the tongue demonstrate displacement and projection.
    *b. everyday memory lapses may be caused by the repression of troubling thoughts and feelings.
    c. painful memories and unacceptable urges will be repressed.
    d. repression is an effective way to deal with troubling thoughts and feelings.

    Page: 276   Topic: Introduction

3. James has forgotten who he is. He does not recognize his wife or his children and has no memory of any events in his life before he regained consciousness in the hospital last week. What category of disorders is James experiencing?
    a. somatoform
    b. psychosomatic
    *c. dissociative
    d. dysfunctional

    Page: 277   Topic: Introduction

4. Alyssa, who is unable to walk, spends her days sitting in a wheelchair. The physicians have found no physical cause for her paralysis. Alyssa is suffering from a _____ disorder.
    a. dissociative
    b. psychotic
    c. psychosomatic
    *d. somatoform

    Page: 227   Topic: Introduction

5. Although he didn't want to do it, Mauricio agreed to conduct a workshop on motivation because he felt pressured by his boss. The day of the workshop, Mauricio called his boss to say he had a fever and chills and would not be able to conduct the workshop. In truth, Mauricio was feeling just fine. In terms of psychological classifications, this is
    *a. malingering.
    b. a factitious disorder.
    c. dissociation.
    d. a somatoform disorder.

    Page: 277   Topic: Introduction

6. In the case study of Helen Fairchild, Dr. McLean noted that Helen's somatic complaint of stomachache and her memory gaps about her childhood may indicate
   a. cognitive deficit.
   *b. childhood sexual abuse.
   c. neurological damage.
   d. satanic rituals.

   Page: 350   Topic: Document 7.1: Dr. Dorothy McLean's Assessment and Preliminary Treatment Plan for Helen Fairchild

7. In her courtroom testimony in the case against Stanley Fairchild for the rape and murder of his daughter's friend, Dr. McLean stated that Helen Fairchild showed signs of all of the following EXCEPT
   a. depersonalization.
   b. somatoform disorder.
   *c. dissociative identity disorder.
   d. dissociative amnesia.

   Page: 282   Topic: Document 7.5: Transcript of Dr. Dorothy McLean's Testimony at the Trial of Stanley Fairchild

8. The text suggests that the psychological disorders of the late 19th century in which people suddenly lost all or part of their memories, dramatically changed personalities, or both
   a. were proven to be hoaxes.
   b. have been recategorized.
   c. vanished.
   *d. went out of style.

   Page: 284   Topic: Amnesia and Fugue

9. Henry remembers events that have occurred since he woke up in the hospital, but he cannot remember events that happened before he was shot. Henry has _____ amnesia.
   *a. retrograde
   b. anterograde
   c. historical
   d. hysterical

   Page: 284   Topic: Amnesia and Fugue

10. According to the text, generalized retrograde amnesia
    a. is the most common type of dissociative disorder.
    *b. occurs more frequently in Hollywood movies than in real life.
    c. is for specific traumatic events.
    d. most commonly occurs when there has been both physical and emotional trauma.

    Page: 284   Topic: Amnesia and Fugue

11. Gregory wandered away from home one day and did not return. His wife, Sara, hired investigators to find him, and, after 3 months, he was located in San Francisco. When Sara approached him and said, "Gregory, please come home," he seemed confused and said, "My name is Sam. Who in the world are you?" Assuming he truly had no memory of his identity or his past, Gregory would be suffering from
    a. factitious disorder.
    b. malingering.
    *c. dissociative fugue.
    d. dissociative identity disorder.

    Page: 284   Topic: Amnesia and Fugue

12. All of the symptoms associated with dissociative amnesia and fugue may also be produced by
    a. vitamin deficiencies.
    b. depression.
    c. hormonal changes.
    *d. organic brain syndromes.

    Page: 285   Topic: Amnesia and Fugue

13. Nelson drinks coffee when he studies and before he goes to class. He says that it helps keep him alert and helps him remember better what he is studying. Based on the literature, the notion of _____ would suggest that Nelson should drink coffee before he takes his exams.
    *a. state-dependent learning
    b. mnemonics
    c. learning dependence
    d. memory techniques

    Page: 286   Topic: Etiology and Treatment of Amnesia and Fugue

14. Therapy for fugue is generally aimed at
    a. helping the person regain his or her identity.
    *b. preventing future episodes.
    c. restoring memories during the fugue state.
    d. helping the person reunite with his or her family.

    Page: 286   Topic: Etiology and Treatment of Amnesia and Fugue

15. In the case study of Helen Fairchild, she told Dr. McLean, "I think I'm going crazy. . . . It's like I'm dreaming even when I'm awake. . . . I can see myself as if I were another person. I'm outside myself, and I can see my face, my hair." These symptoms would meet most of the criteria for
    a. dissociative fugue.
    b. dissociative identity disorder.
    *c. depersonalization disorder.
    d. depressive disorder.

    Pages: 286–287   Topic: Depersonalization Disorder

16. Jeremiah belongs to a religious group in which members regularly fall into trances. However, Jeremiah believes he is possessed, and his behavior differs markedly from other members of his religious group. The diagnosis currently being considered for inclusion in the next edition of the *DSM* to describe this behavior is
    a. depersonalization disorder.
    b. ritualistic disorder.
    c. possession disorder.
    *d. dissociative trance disorder.

    Page: 287   Topic: Depersonalization Disorder

17. Which criterion for depersonalization disorder presents a major diagnostic challenge?
    a. Persistent or recurrent experiences of feeling detached from, and as if one is an outside observer of, one's mental processes or body.
    b. During depersonalization, reality testing remains intact.
    c. The depersonalization causes clinically significant distress or impairment in social, occupational, or other important areas of functioning.
    *d. The depersonalization is not exclusively part of another disorder, a general medical condition, or substance abuse.

    Page: 287   Topic: Depersonalization Disorder

18. The modern era in the study of "multiple personality" (dissociative identity disorder) began in
    a. 1896, when Robert Louis Stevenson published *The Strange Case of Doctor Jekyll and Mr. Hyde.*
    *b. 1908, when Morton Prince published *The Dissociation of a Personality.*
    c. 1954, when Corbett Thigpen and Hervey Cleckley published *The Three Faces of Eve.*
    d. 1975, when Flora Schreiber wrote *Sybil.*

    Page: 288   Topic: Dissociative Identity Disorder

19. According to the text, clinicians' claims that the alternative personalities of a person with dissociative identity disorder can differ physiologically
    a. have demonstrated the strong link between the mind and the body.
    b. have been demonstrated in controlled studies.
    *c. are equivocal at best.
    d. should be included as one of the diagnostic criteria.

    Page: 289   Topic: Diagnosis of Dissociative Identity Disorder

20. All of the following may be "telltale signs" of dissociative identity disorder EXCEPT
    a. findings letters in one's own handwriting, but not remembering writing them.
    b. having headaches and blackouts.
    c. referring to oneself by different names or as "we."
    *d. having fits of rage.

    Page: 289   Topic: Diagnosis of Dissociative Identity Disorder

21. The incidence of dissociative identity disorder
    *a. has been rising over the past 50 years.
    b. has been relatively consistent for the past 50 years.
    c. has been declining over the past 50 years.
    d. goes up and down, depending on societal and environmental events.

    Page: 290   Topic: Is Dissociative Identity Disorder Becoming More Common?

22. Because of the similarity in symptoms, it is possible that some people who meet today's *DSM-IV* diagnostic criteria for dissociative identity disorder would have been diagnosed with which disorder in the past?
    a. major depression
    *b. schizophrenia
    c. depersonalization disorder
    d. post-traumatic stress disorder

    Page: 291   Topic: Is Dissociative Identity Disorder Becoming More Common?

23. An early childhood experience that is connected to dissociative identity disorder is
    a. parents' divorce.
    b. having imaginary playmates.
    *c. childhood sexual abuse.
    d. serious illness.

    Page: 291   Topic: Is Dissociative Identity Disorder Becoming More Common?

24. In assessing Kenneth Bianchi's defense that an alternative personality committed the heinous crimes with which he was charged, psychiatrist Martin Orne testified that
    a. the battery of tests given to Bianchi and the interviews with him supported the claim.
    b. Bianchi was attempting to fool John Watkins, the psychologist who hypnotized him.
    c. Bianchi was suffering from schizophrenia, not dissociative identity disorder.
    *d. Bianchi was faking.

    Page: 291   Topic: Highlight 7.1: Is Dissociative Identity Disorder Real?

25. In the past, psychodynamic therapy treated dissociative identity disorder by
    *a. picking one of the personalities and focusing on that personality's memories.
    b. attempting to fuse the various personalities into a single one.
    c. using drugs such as Amytal and Pentothal Sodium.
    d. teaching coping skills to help the person deal with stress.

    Pages: 291 and 293   Topic: Etiology and Treatment of Dissociative Identity Disorder

26. The unifying theme for the somatoform disorders is that they are
    a. unconcerned with physical symptoms.
    *b. physical manifestations of psychological problems.
    c. psychological manifestations of physical problems.
    d. unique to industrialized countries.

    Page: 294   Topic: Somatoform Disorders

27. William Harvey, physician to King James I, reported the case of a young woman who falsely believed that she was pregnant. The woman was diagnosed with
    a. schizophrenia.
    b. delusional disorder.
    *c. hysteria.
    d. dementia.

    Page: 294   Topic: Conversion Disorder

28. According to Freud, hysterical paralysis of the hand may be
    a. an unconscious desire to avoid distasteful work.
    b. a cry for attention.
    c. a symbolic representation of guilt over wishing someone's death.
    *d. a symbolic representation of guilt over masturbation.

    Page: 294   Topic: Conversion Disorder

29. Conversion disorders may include all of the following EXCEPT
    *a. sexual symptoms.
    b. paralysis.
    c. blindness and deafness.
    d. tingling sensations and anesthesias.

    Page: 294   Topic: Conversion Disorder

30. People with conversion symptoms typically
    a. exhibit *la belle indifference.*
    *b. are troubled by their symptoms.
    c. demonstrate a lack of concern about their symptoms.
    d. fluctuate between concern and lack of concern about their symptoms.

    Page: 294   Topic: Conversion Disorder

31. Slater and Glithero (1965) illustrated the confusion between medical disorders and conversion disorder by following up on people who had been diagnosed with conversion symptoms. They found that on follow-up
    a. 60% of those who had been diagnosed with a medical disorder actually had conversion disorder.
    b. 60% of those who had been diagnosed with conversion disorder also had a medical disorder.
    *c. 60% of those who had been diagnosed with conversion disorder either had died or had been diagnosed with a medical disorder.
    d. the practitioners were almost 100% accurate in their initial diagnoses.

    Page: 294   Topic: Conversion Disorder

32. The modern view of the term *unconscious* refers to
    a. a repository for psychic energy and conflicts.
    b. a person's being in a resting state.
    c. a person's being in a comatose state.
    *d. perceptual and cognitive processes that take place out of awareness.

    Page: 295   Topic: Highlight 7.2: Separating Conversion from Somatic Symptoms

33. Hillary woke up terrified one morning. She told her husband she could not see anything—she was blind. Her husband immediately made an appointment with her ophthalmologist, who examined Hillary's eyes. Upon finishing the examination, the doctor began to walk out of the room, then turned to Hillary and asked her to follow him to another room. Since Hillary was able to avoid obstacles that had been placed on the floor of the room, the doctor determined that Hillary
    *a. had hysterical blindness.
    b. was faking it.
    c. had developed a keen sense of kinesthetics.
    d. had macular degeneration.

    Page: 295   Topic: Highlight 7.2: Separating Conversion from Somatic Symptoms

34. How do psychoanalytic psychologists explain the decrease in the prevalence of conversion disorders?
    a. Conversion disorders have become "unfashionable" in today's world.
    *b. Today's more open attitudes toward sex have eliminated the main cause of conversion disorders.
    c. Conversion disorders were primarily diagnosed in women, and as women gain more power, they no longer need the disorder.
    d. Due to improved diagnostic techniques, symptoms that were previously diagnosed as conversion disorder now receive other diagnoses.

    Page: 296   Topic: Prevalence, Family Patterns, and Course

35. The individual who would be LEAST likely to develop a conversion disorder would be someone
    a. from a rural area.
    b. with a low income.
    *c. with a college education.
    d. who belongs to a fundamentalist religion.

    Page: 297   Topic: Prevalence, Family Patterns, and Course

36. After an emotionally devastating argument with her husband, Melanie developed conversion hysteria in the form of muteness. Her husband is now totally repentant, and she is receiving a great deal of attention and support from her family and friends. Her psychoanalyst is most likely to focus Melanie's treatment on
    a. reducing the secondary gain Melanie receives by way of attention from others.
    b. encouraging Melanie's family and friends (and especially her husband) to provide her with even more support.
    c. encouraging Melanie to communicate nonverbally until she is again able to express herself verbally.
    *d. uncovering and showing how conflicts contribute to the muteness and helping Melanie express her psychological needs in a better way.

    Page: 298   Topic: Etiology and Treatment

37. On the last day of his final exams, Antonio found that he could not move his right hand. A neurological evaluation showed no physical problems. When his friends, family, and professors learned of his condition, they rallied around him and offered support, sympathy, attention, and assistance. All of this attention and help for Antonio would be a

    *a. secondary gain.
    b. primary gain.
    c. tertiary gain.
    d. positive gain.

    Page: 297   Topic: Etiology and Treatment

38. Selena has been unable to walk since the day before her mother's funeral. A battery of neurological tests has shown no organic basis for her paralysis. Which health care professional would we expect Selena to be LEAST likely to seek out to help her with her paralysis?

    a. a neurologist
    *b. a psychologist
    c. an anesthesiologist
    d. an internist

    Page: 298   Topic: Etiology and Treatment

39. Which treatment is MOST likely to help someone suffering from conversion disorder?

    a. psychoanalysis
    b. behaviorism
    *c. bogus medical treatment
    d. real medical treatment

    Page: 298   Topic: Etiology and Treatment

40. Amir has multiple physical complaints, although none of the several physicians he has seen has found any organic basis for these ailments. He complains of chest pains, pains in his abdomen and back, headaches, nausea, bloating, erectile dysfunction, and double vision. These symptoms are significantly affecting his ability to work and maintain his relationship. Amir would most likely be diagnosed with

    a. conversion disorder.
    b. hypochondriasis.
    c. pain disorder.
    *d. somatization disorder.

    Page: 298   Topic: Somatization Disorder

41. Pearl was in the hospital, insisting that she be treated for a multiplicity of medical problems, even though none of her doctors could find a medical basis for her complaints. However, while she was in the hospital, she developed tuberculosis and blood poisoning, which ultimately killed her. Pearl finally succumbed to _____ disorder.

    *a. an iatrogenic
    b. a somatization
    c. a conversion
    d. an undifferentiated somatoform

    Page: 299   Topic: Somatization Disorder

42. Linda complained of dizziness, paralysis, and strange sensory phenomena that would come and go. Because she was under extreme stress, the doctor thought she might have somatization disorder, but Linda's symptoms also require that _____ be ruled out as well.
   a. Crohn's disease
   *b. multiple sclerosis
   c. chronic fatigue syndrome
   d. muscular dystrophy

   Page: 299   Topic: Somatization Disorder

43. Muriel was seen in a psychiatric clinic, presenting with impaired memory or concentration, sore throat, tender lymph nodes, muscle pain, joint pain, headaches, and irregular sleep patterns (insomnia at night, inability to stay awake during the day). Considering the symptoms and the setting, Muriel would most likely be diagnosed as having
   a. conversion hysteria.
   b. chronic fatigue syndrome.
   *c. somatization disorder.
   d. Crohn's disease.

   Page: 299   Topic: Critical Thinking About . . . 7.1: Mind Versus Body: The Case of Chronic Fatigue
                Syndrome

44. In what way do diagnoses for somatization disorder differ for men and women?
   a. They do not differ; the prevalence rate is the same for both.
   b. Due to their higher estrogen levels, women are less likely than men to succumb to these disorders.
   c. The differences are actually between cultures (higher frequency in less industrialized nations), not between genders.
   *d. Men are less likely to be diagnosed with these disorders because, in some cultures, it is not considered "masculine" to complain about being sick.

   Page: 300   Topic: Prevalence, Family Patterns, and Course

45. When men have somatization disorder, they are more likely than women to exhibit all of the following EXCEPT
   *a. medical complaints.
   b. alcohol abuse.
   c. drug abuse.
   d. criminal activity.

   Page: 301   Topic: Etiology and Treatment

46. Adoption studies indicate that somatization disorders are most likely due to
   a. heredity.
   *b. environmental factors.
   c. genetics.
   d. trauma.

   Page: 301   Topic: Etiology and Treatment

47. Dr. Allen is treating Soon-Yi for somatization disorder. He is using a technique called response prevention, which
    a. encourages Soon-Yi to talk about her childhood, but prohibits her from talking about her imagined illness.
    b. involves free association and dream interpretation, which Dr. Allen immediately relates to Soon-Yi's past when she begins to talk about her imagined illness.
    *c. keeps Soon-Yi from consulting a medical practitioner for her imagined illness.
    d. encourages Soon-Yi to consult a medical practitioner for her imagined illness as well as for other ailments she does not actually experience.

    Page: 301   Topic: Etiology and Treatment

48. Dr. Ellis, a cognitive therapist, is treating Gloria for somatization disorder. Dr. Ellis is likely to do all of the following EXCEPT
    a. get Gloria to accept responsibility for her behavior.
    b. teach Gloria the skills she needs to cope with anxiety more adaptively.
    c. teach Gloria the skills she needs to cope with frustration more adaptively.
    *d. confront Gloria with the psychological nature of her problems.

    Page: 301   Topic: Etiology and Treatment

49. Pain disorder would be diagnosed when
    *a. psychological factors are dominant in the pain.
    b. the pain is related to sexual intercourse.
    c. the pain from an injury or illness has become chronic.
    d. pain is combined with other somatic symptoms.

    Page: 302   Topic: Pain Disorder

50. Aisha obsesses over her health, although she appears not to have any specific physical symptoms. She is always disappointed when her doctors say they can find nothing wrong with her. Aisha most likely has
    a. somatization disorder.
    *b. hypochondriasis.
    c. conversion disorder.
    d. obsessive-compulsive disorder.

    Page: 304   Topic: Hypochondriasis

51. For centuries, hypochondriasis was considered to be
    a. an unfindable medical disorder.
    b. a disorder that only women got.
    *c. the male form of hysteria.
    d. associated with the menstrual cycle.

    Page: 303   Topic: Hypochondriasis

52. All of the following are typical of hypochondriacs EXCEPT:
    a. they misinterpret normal bodily symptoms.
    b. they fear a particular disease rather than just symptoms.
    c. their disorder exacts a severe toll on their family and social life.
    *d. they use the disorder to avoid work or family responsibilities.

    Page: 304   Topic: Hypochondriasis

53. Our knowledge of etiology and treatment outcome for hypochondriacs is based on
    *a. the small number of atypical hypochondriacal people who agree to participate in psychological research and attend psychological clinics.
    b. the large number of typical hypochondriacal people who agree to participate in psychological research and attend psychological clinics.
    c. the large number of typical hypochondriacal people who refuse psychological treatment, but persistently seek medical treatment.
    d. survey research from persons assumed to have hypochondriasis (from their responses), as well as friends and relatives of hypochondriacs.

    Page: 304   Topic: Etiology and Treatment

54. Dr. Jerome believes that people with hypochondriasis have a tendency to attribute serious illness to benign symptoms. This phenomenon is known as
    a. attributional process.
    *b. somatosensory amplification.
    c. irrational thought process.
    d. symptom amplification.

    Page: 305   Topic: Etiology and Treatment

55. In their research on hypochondriasis, Hitchcock and Mathews (1992) found that
    a. college students are more likely to be hypochondriacs than are those who are not currently in school.
    b. previous severe illness or physical trauma (such as broken bones) seems to predispose people to hypochondria.
    *c. hypochondriacs tend to attribute their pains to serious underlying diseases.
    d. hypochondriacs tend to attribute their pains to some type of injury, but they attribute other symptoms to underlying diseases.

    Page: 305   Topic: Etiology and Treatment

56. Barbie has had 37 cosmetic surgeries to various parts of her body in order to make her the most beautiful woman in the world. She began once she graduated from high school, and she anticipates at least 10 more surgeries before she will be what she considers "perfect." She has a Web site on the Internet to give advice to other people who are thinking of undergoing surgery. Barbie is suffering from
    a. anorexia nervosa.
    b. obsessive-compulsive disorder.
    c. factitious disorder.
    *d. body dysmorphic disorder.

    Page: 305   Topic: Body Dysmorphic Disorder

57. Baron von Klaus persistently lies about his health, always saying that he had one horrible disease or another. He describes his illnesses in dramatic terms, using medical jargon, and seems to take great joy in being ill. He also takes great pride in discussing the many times he has been hospitalized for diseases the doctors could not find. Most likely von Klaus is suffering from
    *a. a factitious disorder.
    b. malingering.
    c. hypochondriasis.
    d. Munchausen by proxy.

    Page: 307   Topic: Factitious Disorders

58. Bartlett's (1950) research with memory demonstrates that
   a. our memories are very poor.
   *b. memories are reconstructed in light of our own experiences.
   c. memories can be reconstructed depending on questions that are asked.
   d. memories can be easily manipulated.

   Page: 310   Topic: Recovered Memories May Be Inaccurate

59. The guidelines issued by the professional groups around the world that deal with people in psychological treatment
   a. indicate a great distrust of recovered memories of childhood abuse.
   b. require that any alleged recovered memories of childhood abuse be corroborated by third parties.
   *c. recognize that memories of early child abuse may be forgotten, but remembered later in life.
   d. state that alleged recovered memories should be explored only if doing so will not harm others in the event the memories are false.

   Page: 311   Topic: Ethical Responsibilities

60. In the case study of Helen Fairchild, the defense attorney
   a. acknowledged the fact that Helen was sexually abused but denied that she could have remembered her father murdering her friend.
   b. accused Helen of concocting the story about her father murdering her friend in order to get back at him for years of sexual abuse.
   c. accused Helen of concocting all aspects of the case against her father, including the sexual abuse and the murder of Helen's friend.
   *d. accused the therapist of taking a vulnerable woman (Helen) and planting false memories of murder and abuse.

   Page: 313   Topic: Document 7.10: Excerpt from the Summation for the Defense

TRUE-FALSE QUESTIONS

61. Freud believed that there is a continuity between what is normal and what is abnormal. (T)

   Page: 276   Topic: Introduction

62. According to Freud, repression is an abnormal process aimed at keeping thoughts out of conscious awareness. (F)

   Page: 276   Topic: Introduction

63. Almost all cases of dissociative amnesia are of the retrograde type. (T)

   Page: 284   Topic: Amnesia and Fugue

64. Most people who suffer from dissociative fugue move to another town, assume a new name, start a new job, and change their personalities. (F)

   Page: 285   Topic: Amnesia and Fugue

65. In contrast to people with a depersonalization disorder, people with schizophrenia may experience some of the same symptoms, but those with depersonalization disorder lose touch with reality. (F)

   Page: 287   Topic: Depersonalization Disorder

66. Practically every aspect of dissociative identity disorder is the subject of intense controversy. (T)

   Page: 288   Topic: Dissociative Identity Disorder

67. The use of hypnosis in assessing dissociative identity disorder ensures the legitimacy of a diagnosis. (F)

   Page: 290   Topic: Is Dissociative Identity Disorder Becoming More Common?

68. Psychologists have developed highly sensitive techniques for judging whether someone is, in fact, faking dissociative identity disorder. (F)

Page: 291   Topic: Is Dissociative Identity Disorder Becoming More Common?

69. Amytal and Pentothal Sodium have been used to get people with dissociative identity disorder to reveal their repressed memories. (T)

Page: 293   Topic: Etiology and Treatment of Dissociative Identity Disorder

70. Controlled outcome studies of treatments for dissociative identity disorder indicate that early diagnosis predicts a poor prognosis. (F)

Page: 293   Topic: Etiology and Treatment of Dissociative Identity Disorder

71. High-technology laboratory tests and expensive diagnostic equipment for determining whether symptoms are somatic are often insufficient to determine whether symptoms are due to a medical problem. (T)

Page: 295   Topic: Highlight 7.2: Separating Conversion from Somatic Symptoms

72. Men are more likely than women to be diagnosed with a conversion disorder. (F)

Page: 296   Topic: Prevalence, Family Patterns, and Course

73. The consistency between the *DSM* and the *ICD* makes it relatively easy to compare diagnoses cross-culturally. (F)

Page: 297   Topic: Prevalence, Family Patterns, and Course

74. Significant evidence for a genetic factor in conversion disorders has not been found. (T)

Page: 297   Topic: Etiology and Treatment

75. People with somatization disorder repeat the same story about their medical history to each and every doctor they see. (F)

Page: 299   Topic: Somatization Disorder

76. Somatoform disorders support the position that sees a rigid distinction between mind and body. (F)

Page: 299   Topic: Somatization Disorder

77. It is difficult to estimate the lifetime prevalence of somatization disorder because each version of the *DSM* has used different diagnostic criteria. (T)

Page: 299   Topic: Prevalence, Family Patterns, and Course

78. Most people who have pain disorder also have other medical and psychological disorders. (T)

Page: 302   Topic: Pain Disorder

79. Unlike psychological disorders, which come and go and are ever changing, medical diseases are persistent over time. (F)

Pages: 303–304   Topic: Hyponchondriasis

80. Recovered memories of abuse have often been independently verified. (T)

Page: 310   Topic: Recovered Memories May Be Accurate

SHORT-ANSWER QUESTIONS

81. Differentiate between anterograde amnesia and retrograde amnesia.

    With anterograde amnesia, sufferers can remember events that occurred before a traumatic experience, but new events are forgotten shortly after they occur. With retrograde amnesia, events that took place before a traumatic event are forgotten, but sufferers remember events that happened after the trauma.

    Page: 284   Topic: Amnesia and Fugue

82. Describe the four clinical signs that may help to distinguish organic from dissociative amnesia and fugues.

    Organic amnesias usually result from degenerative diseases that develop gradually, whereas dissociative amnesias come on suddenly; organic amnesias are typically anterograde, whereas dissociative amnesias are almost always retrograde; dissociative amnesia is associated with severe psychological stress; and people with organic amnesias do not usually take on new identities.

    Pages: 284–286   Topic: Amnesia and Fugue

83. What are the criteria for a diagnosis of dissociative identity disorder?

    Presence of two or more distinct identities or personality states (each with its own relatively enduring pattern of perceiving, relating to, and thinking about the environment or self); at least two of these identities or personality states recurrently taking control of the person's behavior; inability to recall important personal information that is too extensive to be explained by ordinary forgetfulness; and the disturbance is not due to the direct physiological effects of a substance or a general medical condition (in children, the symptoms are not due to imaginary playmates or fantasy play).

    Page: 289   Topic: Table 7.5: Main *DSM-IV* Diagnostic Criteria for Dissociative Identity Disorder

84. What factors does the text suggest are involved in the development of dissociative identity disorder?

    child sexual abuse, physical abuse, susceptibility to "self-hypnosis"

    Page: 290   Topic: Is Dissociative Identity Disorder Becoming More Common?

85. What are the five somatoform disorders described in the *DSM-IV?*

    conversion disorder, somatization disorder, pain disorder, hypochondriasis, body dysmorphic disorder

    Page: 293   Topic: Somatoform Disorders

86. How would psychoanalytic psychologists explain the decrease in the prevalence of conversion disorders and the expected gender differences in the expression of these disorders?

    Freud's turn-of-the-century Vienna was sexually inhibited, and today's more open attitudes toward sex have eliminated the main cause of conversion disorders. Because the few sexual taboos that remain today apply more to women than to men, we should expect a higher prevalence of conversion disorders among women than men, which is, indeed, the case.

    Page: 296   Topic: Prevalence, Family Patterns, and Course

87. What factors would characterize someone who is most likely to develop a conversion disorder?

    being from a rural area, with little education, a low income, and a fundamentalist religious background; or being from a developing society; or being a newcomer to the United States.

    Page: 372   Topic: Prevalence, Family Patterns, and Course

88. Describe the suspicious signs that may alert clinicians to the possibility of a somatization disorder.

    Complaints that span biological systems (gastrointestinal, neurological, respiratory) are suspect because there are relatively few medical conditions that affect multiple organ systems; and complaints that last for decades without any deterioration or improvement.

    Page: 299   Topic: Somatization Disorder

89. Discuss the cultural differences seen in somatization disorder.

The disorder is more common among Chinese Americans than Caucasian Americans, and it is especially common in India. Reports of "feeling as if worms are crawling under the skin" are common in Africa but hardly ever encountered in the United States or Europe. Across cultures, somatic symptoms are correlated with emotional distress: The greater the distress, the higher the number of symptoms reported by both males and females.

Page: 301   Topic: Prevalence, Family Patterns, and Course

90. What are the various factors involved in a person's response to pain, and how do they affect treatment?

A person's response to pain is a complicated function of tissue damage, social background, personality, coping skills, and social supports. Successful treatment often requires a combination of physiological and psychological interventions.

Page: 302   Topic: Pain Disorder

91. Discuss the prevalence factors noted with regard to hypochondriasis.

Prevalence estimates range from 3% to 13%, with equal numbers of men and women affected; the disorder is not closely related to education, social class, or ethnicity, nor is it strongly correlated with age. It is a chronic condition that waxes and wanes but never completely disappears.

Pages: 302–303   Topic: Hypochondriasis

92. Describe the characteristics of people with body dysmorphic disorder.

They are obsessed with supposed defects in their appearance: Defects such as hair loss, skin blemishes, scars, the shape of their nose, the size of their breasts, etc., which are either imaginary or highly exaggerated, become the focus of concern. They may give up social commitments and stay away from work to avoid being seen, and in severe cases, social isolation becomes so extreme that they see suicide as the only way out.

Page: 305   Topic: Body Dysmorphic Disorder

93. Differentiate between malingering and factitious disorders.

People with both fake their symptoms, but malingerers have a clear reason for doing so, such as avoiding responsibilities, providing evidence for a lawsuit, or keeping fed and warm for the winter. Malingering may be adaptive, such as in hostages who pretend to be sick to escape from their captors. Those with factitious disorders receive no obvious reward other than attention.

Pages: 307–309   Topic: Factitious Disorders

94. Discuss the "two sides" of the recovered memory debate.

There is clear evidence that traumatic events can be pushed out of consciousness, and that long-forgotten memories may come flooding back in psychotherapy; there is also evidence of large numbers of cases of child sexual abuse. However, memories are affected by a person's experience, and memories can be affected by the types of questions asked. The underlying question is whether therapists can actually "plant" memories for events that never took place.

Pages: 309–311   Topic: Recovered Memories

95. What do psychotherapeutic guidelines state about how psychologists should act in cases where memories may be recovered?

   They recognize that memories of early child abuse may sometimes be forgotten, only to be remembered much later in life; they admit that it is possible to recover memories of early-childhood abuse. However, they also recognize that individuals may sometimes construct memories of early abuse that seem real to them but that never happened. Mental health professionals should be aware of the constructive nature of memory, of the potential for leading questions and suggestions to distort memory, and that hypnosis or drugs do not make memory any more or less accurate. Thus, ethical therapists should never suggest to clients that they were abused but should adopt a neutral stance in gathering information.

   Pages: 311–312   Topic: Ethical Responsibilities

ESSAY QUESTIONS

96. Your professor has asked the class whether Helen Fairchild, the case study in this chapter, suffered from a dissociative, somatoform, or factitious disorder. Different students have taken various positions, and you have been asked to sum it all up. Address each of the disorders in terms of Helen Fairchild's case.

   This will involve a discussion not only of the various forms of each of these disorders, but also of how they apply to the case in the text.

97. As you enter the library, you hear loud voices coming from one of the study rooms. You walk over to see what's going on and find three of your classmates in heated debate. They tell you they're arguing about the role of unconscious thoughts and feelings in the dissociative, somatoform, and factitious disorders. One states that it's so obvious, you can watch even normal people and see how these processes play out, the second says it's all a matter of learning, and the third shouts over them that these disorders come out of people's irrational thoughts. They ask you what you think of each of their positions. Explain your position.

   Discuss how the psychoanalytic, behavioral, and cognitive-behavioral approaches explain each of these disorders.

98. Knowing you are taking this class in abnormal psychology, your next-door neighbor approaches you and asks for advice. She tells you her whole family is a bit "off" and goes on to explain what she means. As you listen to her, you learn that within her immediate and extended families there can be found most of the disorders discussed in this chapter. When she finishes, she asks you what type of therapy you think would be most successful in helping these people she dearly loves. What would you suggest?

   This requires a discussion not only of the various types of therapy that have been used—including placebos—for the different disorders, but also an understanding that, particularly with the somatoform and factitious disorders, there will be resistance to the suggestion that the disorders are, in any way, psychological. Further, in light of the whole family's being involved, there should be a focus on family therapy.

99. A startling case is spread across the news media—on television and radio, in newspapers and magazines. The case involves a woman who claims to have been sexually abused by her father, her father's brother, and her own brother when she was a child. All three have denied the abuse and are suing the woman's psychologist for "planting false memories." Based on what you have read in the chapter, what symptoms would you expect to see in this woman? What evidence do you believe would support her allegations? What issues would you need to consider in deciding whether the memories are real or were created by way of suggestion?

   Address the somatic and behavioral symptoms that would suggest child sexual abuse; then discuss both sides of the false memory debate.

100. One of your friends has recently joined a support group for survivors of sexual abuse. A woman in the group confided that she had no memory of her abuse until she began reading books about child sexual abuse and considered the behavioral manifestations that are likely to result from such early trauma. She then started to have vague flashbacks that troubled her, so she went to see a therapist. The therapist suggested that her symptoms were consistent with child sexual abuse and, in addition to ongoing therapy, encouraged the woman to join this group. Your friend asks you about the ethical issues involved in delving into a person's past. What could you tell her?

The two important issues here are the psychotherapeutic approach taken (the psychoanalytic approach, of course, will delve into the past) and how the information is elicited from the client (the care the therapist takes to avoid making statements or asking questions in a way that will elicit information that didn't happen from a client who is attempting to please the therapist).

CHAPTER 8
THE MOOD DISORDER SPECTRUM: FROM THE BLUES TO DEPRESSIVE AND BIPOLAR DISORDERS

MULTIPLE-CHOICE QUESTIONS

1. Depression is categorized as _____ disorder.
   *a.   a mood
   b.   a dissociative
   c.   an anxiety
   d.   a personality

   Page: 318   Topic: Introduction

2. Jack is "on top of the world." He is so excited that, after 72 hours of work at his computer with no rest, he has written a magnificent treatise on world peace. He now has charged airline flights on his credit card so that he can visit the heads of state of the major world nations to share his brilliant plan with them. His energy is unbounded. In terms of the mood disorders, Jack most likely is experiencing
   a.   dysphoria.
   *b.   mania.
   c.   an obsession.
   d.   dysthymia.

   Page: 318   Topic: Introduction

3. Clinicians will suspect the presence of a mood disorder when:
   a.   a client tells them that she is "down" after graduating with honors.
   b.   a client expresses grief over the breakup of a relationship.
   *c.   a negative mood persists and affects social and occupational functioning.
   d.   a positive mood persists despite negative environmental experiences.

   Page: 319   Topic: Introduction

4. In the classic television and movie series *Star Trek,* Dr. McCoy often accuses Mr. Spock of being _____ because Spock lacks the ability to feel emotions.
   a   an excellent leader
   b.   intellectual
   c.   intelligent
   *d.   inhuman

   Page: 320   Topic: Emotions: Normal and Pathological

5. Charles Darwin hypothesized that emotions evolved because
   *a.   they have survival value.
   b.   our brains became more complex than the brains of other animals.
   c.   we modeled the behavior of other social animals.
   d.   they allow us to express our innermost thoughts.

   Page: 320   Topic: Emotions: Normal and Pathological

6. Sorrow has survival value in that it
    a. helps people bond with others, keeping them safe by ensuring that others will be around.
    *b. keeps parents close to their children, increasing their offspring's chances of survival.
    c. balances out joyous emotions, providing equilibrium for the nervous system.
    d. allows us to value our elders and our ancestors, ensuring we will care for those who hold knowledge and wisdom.

    Page: 320   Topic: Emotions: Normal and Pathological

7. _____ an important determinant of how quickly, and how well, people cope with the grieving process.
    a. Rituals are
    *b. Social support is
    c. Solitude is
    d. Religious proscriptions are

    Page: 321   Topic: Grieving

8. Audrey has been diagnosed with dysthymic disorder. This is
    a. an extreme form of depression.
    b. a combination of depression and mania.
    *c. a relatively mild condition.
    d. another name for depression.

    Page: 321   Topic: *DSM-IV* Mood Disorders

9. All of the following are bipolar disorders EXCEPT
    a. bipolar I.
    b. bipolar II.
    c. cyclothymic disorder.
    *d. dysthymic disorder.

    Page: 321   Topic: *DSM-IV* Mood Disorders

10. In the Golden Age of Greece, melancholia was associated with _____ bile.
    *a. black
    b. white
    c. yellow
    d. red

    Page: 321   Topic: Depressive (Unipolar) Disorders

11. Which Biblical figure has been recorded as suffering from melancholy?
    a. King David
    *b. King Saul
    c. the prophet Jeremiah
    d. Abraham

    Page: 321   Topic: Depressive (Unipolar) Disorders

12. The most famous book ever written about depression was written by
    a. Hippocrates.
    b. Sigmund Freud.
    *c. Robert Burton.
    d. Martin E. P. Seligman.

    Page: 321   Topic: Depressive (Unipolar) Disorders

13. Maria's boyfriend broke off their five-year relationship. For the first five months after the breakup, Maria went through periods of extreme sadness, and she constantly doubted her ability to do even the simplest of things. She saw herself as a loser who was not worthy of being loved. By the sixth month, however, the periods of sadness began to come less often, and she started to regain her self-confidence. According to the *DSM-IV*, Maria experienced
    a. normal grieving.
    b. dysthymia.
    c. a temporary major depressive disorder.
    *d. adjustment disorder with depressive features.

    Pages: 322–323   Topic: Major Depressive Episode: Signs

14. The inability to feel pleasure, as seen in major depression, is termed
    *a. anhedonia.
    b. emotional anesthesia.
    c. aphasia.
    d. morbidity.

    Page: 322   Topic: Major Depressive Episode: Signs

15. Claudine saw no reason to get up in the morning. Life was dull, she felt apathetic and sad, and she no longer found pleasure in doing the things she used to find enjoyable. Her thoughts had slowed down to what she described as "almost a stop." Claudine appears to be experiencing
    a. an adjustment disorder with depressive features.
    *b. a major depressive episode.
    c. bipolar disorder.
    d. a dysthymic episode.

    Pages: 322–323   Topic: Major Depressive Episode: Signs

16. Which of the following thoughts would be most consistent with a major depressive episode?
    a. "I'm not very good at math, so I'd better study harder."
    b. "Everything's going wrong today. Maybe if I go to bed, things will be better when I wake up."
    *c. "I don't blame him for breaking up with me. I'm really unlovable."
    d. "The world is falling apart—there's war everywhere. It's all because of the politicians we vote into office."

    Page: 323   Topic: Major Depressive Episode: Signs

17. "Anger attacks," the sudden, intense spells of anger experienced by depressed people that are associated with a surge of autonomic arousal including rapid heart rate, sweating, flushing, and a feeling of being out of control, are related to
    a. changes in their physiological makeup.
    b. hormonal disturbances.
    c. reactions to the negative emotions of the people around them.
    *d. negative cognitions.

    Page: 323   Topic: Major Depressive Episode: Signs

18. Who of the following is the LEAST likely to be experiencing a major depressive episode?
    *a. 5-month-old Tanya, who is always agitated, irritable, and has constant stomachaches
    b. 8-month-old Erica, who is listless and apathetic and does not respond to being cuddled
    c. 2-year-old Jennifer, who has recurrent stomachaches, earaches, sore throats, and pains in her chest
    d. 17-year-old Jessica, who is pessimistic, unmotivated, believes she is worthless, and constantly feels fatigued

    Page: 324   Topic: Major Depressive Episode: Signs

19. Which of the following comorbid relationships is LEAST likely to be seen with major depression?
    a. physical illness and depression
    *b. obsessive-compulsive disorder and depression
    c. substance abuse and depression
    d. generalized anxiety disorder and depression

    Page: 325   Topic: Comorbid Conditions

20. The most widely used assessment device for depression in the United States is the
    a. MMPI.
    b. Depression Self-Rating Scale.
    *c. Beck Depression Inventory.
    d. Brief Depression Rating Scale.

    Page: 325   Topic: Psychological Assessment

21. Major depressive disorder
    a. has more extreme symptoms than does a major depressive episode.
    b. is another name for a major depressive episode.
    c. rarely occurs in those who are diagnosed with a major depressive episode.
    *d. is a chronic condition consisting of one or more major depressive episodes.

    Page: 326   Topic: Major Depressive Disorder

22. Sylvia just lost her job and her husband ran off with her best friend. Sylvia's depression would be categorized as
    *a. exogenous.
    b. endogenous.
    c. exogamous.
    d. endogamous.

    Page: 326   Topic: Major Depressive Disorder

23. Who is likely to spend the most time in bed and have difficulty pursuing her normal activities?
    a. Pearl, who suffers from diabetes
    *b. Cindy, who suffers from major depressive disorder
    c. Aileen, who suffers from arthritis
    d. Rose, who suffers from asthma

    Page: 326   Topic: Major Depressive Disorder

24. Which of the following is true about dysthymia?
    a. It is more serious than depression.
    b. The symptoms may disappear for several months at a time.
    *c. It lasts at least 2 years, but may go on for decades.
    d. A diagnosis requires the presence of at least four depressive symptoms.

    Page: 326   Topic: Dysthymic Disorder

25. Alfredo has been diagnosed with dysthymic disorder as well as occasional major depressive episodes. Alfredo suffers from
    a. major depression.
    b. dysthymia with severe depressive disorder.
    c. dual diagnosis.
    *d. double depression.

    Page: 326   Topic: Dysthymic Disorder

26. The majority of depressed people
    *a. are called "atypical."
    b. are dysthymic.
    c. have major depressive episodes.
    d. have major depressive disorder.

    Page: 326   Topic: Dysthymic Disorder

27. Clinical depression is called the "common cold" of psychological disorders because
    a. there is no known cure.
    *b. so many people get it.
    c. symptoms can be reduced with medication.
    d. symptoms remain for an extended period of time.

    Page: 326   Topic: Prevalence and Course of Depressive Disorders

28. The text implicates all of the following in the increase in depression EXCEPT
    a. the widespread use of psychoactive substances.
    b. mass international migrations.
    *c. ever-increasing technological advances.
    d. the breakdown of the traditional family.

    Page: 326   Topic: Prevalence and Course of Depressive Disorders

29. Compared with its historical appearance, today depression has become a disorder of
    a. older people.
    b. adults.
    c. preadolescents.
    *d. young people.

    Page: 326   Topic: Prevalence and Course of Depressive Disorders

30. Which of the following statements about depression is FALSE?
    *a. Most episodes of depression take several years to improve.
    b. One of the outcomes of the increase in depression among young people is an increase in suicide rates.
    c. Depression is likely to become a more serious problem in the future because it is beginning earlier in life than in years past.
    d. The earlier depression begins, the more likely it is to become chronic.

    Page: 327   Topic: Prevalence and Course of Depressive Disorders

31. Who is MOST likely to develop a depressive disorder?
    a. Jerome, a 30-year-old business executive who works at the corporate office 60 hours a week
    *b. Jeralyn, a 30-year-old homemaker who has two young children and does not work outside the home
    c. Janice, a 25-year-old woman who owns her own architectural firm and has two young children at home
    d. Janay, a 22-year-old woman who will receive her MBA in June but has not yet found the "man of her dreams"

    Page: 328   Topic: Sex, Ethnic, and Cultural Differences

32. In which group is depression equally common in both sexes?
    a. African Americans
    b. Catholics
    *c. the Amish
    d. new immigrants

    Page: 328   Topic: Sex, Ethnic, and Cultural Differences

33. Members of which culture are most likely to express depression in terms of loss of interest in formerly pleasurable activities and feelings of worthlessness?
    a. Latin
    b. Asian
    c. Mediterranean
    *d. northern European

    Page: 328   Topic: Sex, Ethnic, and Cultural Differences

34. The term *bipolar* refers to all of the following EXCEPT
    *a. people whose episodes of dysthymia alternate with episodes of depression.
    b. people whose episodes of elevated mood alternate with periods of depression.
    c. people who display only manic episodes.
    d. manic people whose depressed state has not yet manifested itself.

    Pages: 328–329   Topic: Bipolar Disorders

35. All of the following are characteristics of manic episodes EXCEPT
    a. rapid and unfocused thought
    *b. decreased sex drive
    c. energized and chaotic physical activity
    d. rapid speech and frequent topic switching that produces incoherence

    Page: 330   Topic: Manic, Hypomanic, and Mixed Episodes

36. People who display manic symptoms while having a depressed mood are said to have
    a. double depression.
    b. manic depression.
    *c. a mixed episode.
    d. schizophrenia.

    Page: 330   Topic: Manic, Hypomanic, and Mixed Episodes

37. Hubert appears to be elated and industrious. He is typically in an elated mood, has little need for sleep, and has intense periods of activity. However, he tends to skip from one activity to another, rarely carries his plans to completion, and has a low tolerance for frustration. Because he does not show the extremes of mania, Hubert would be considered to have
    a. a cheery disposition.
    b. a mixed episode.
    c. hypermania.
    *d. hypomania.

    Page: 330   Topic: Manic, Hypomanic, and Mixed Episodes

38. _____ consists of one or more manic or mixed episodes, and, in most cases, individuals will also have had one or more major depressive episodes.
    *a. Bipolar I disorder
    b. Bipolar II disorder
    c. Cyclothymic disorder
    d. Dysthymic disorder

    Page: 331   Topic: Specific Bipolar Disorders

39. _____ involves frequent mood swings in which hypomanic symptoms alternate with symptoms of mild depression over a period of 2 years.
   a. Dysthymic disorder
   *b. Cyclothymic disorder
   c. Bipolar I disorder
   d. Bipolar II disorder

   Page: 331   Topic: Specific Bipolar Disorders

40. Every month, at the same time during each of her menstrual cycles, Cynthia experiences depressed mood. This mood disorder, which is presently being considered for inclusion in the *DSM-V,* is called
   a. postmenstrual syndrome.
   b. premenstrual dysthymic disorder.
   *c. premenstrual dysphoric disorder.
   d. dysthymic disorder.

   Page: 331   Topic: Specific Bipolar Disorders

41. A critical reason for NOT including premenstrual dysphoric disorder in the *DSM* is
   a. that the mental health field is controlled by men.
   b. that it is not recognized as an abnormal condition.
   c. the lack of evidence that the disorder is related to hormonal changes.
   *d. the concern that doing so might perpetuate the stereotype that women's emotions are less controllable than those of men.

   Page: 331   Topic: Specific Bipolar Disorders

42. The most compelling reason to believe that bipolar disorder and major depressive disorder are two distinct conditions is that
   *a. they respond to different treatments.
   b. they have different symptoms.
   c. it is rare that someone is both happy and sad at the same time.
   d. they can be differentiated by their degree of severity.

   Page: 331   Topic: Specific Bipolar Disorders

43. Bipolar disorders are diagnosed more often
   a. in women than in men.
   *b. among members of higher than lower socioeconomic groups.
   c. among younger people than among older people.
   d. among members of ethnic-minority groups than in members of other groups.

   Page: 331   Topic: Prevalence and Course of Bipolar Disorders

44. After 20 years of marriage, Karolyn finally divorced Richard. His mood swings, irritability, grandiose plans that were never completed, and unpredictability were more than she could bear. Unlike others with bipolar disorder, Richard's moods would alternate several times a month. Richard was a
   a. cyclothymic.
   b. hyperthymic.
   *c. rapid cycler.
   d. multi-cycler.

   Page: 332   Topic: Prevalence and Course of Bipolar Disorders

45. Anita consistently becomes extremely depressed during the winter, but as summer approaches, her depression abates. Which specifier would apply to her mood disorder?
   a. postpartum
   b. melancholic
   c. catatonic
   *d. seasonal

   Page: 332   Topic: Diagnostic Specifiers

46. The first step in studies addressing the etiology of mood disorders is to
   *a. diagnose probands using specified criteria and structured interviews.
   b. look for relatives of people who have mood disorders.
   c. interview and evaluate the family members of people who have mood disorders.
   d. assess the social settings and hereditary influences of people with mood disorders.

   Page: 334   Topic: Genetics

47. Twin studies have found that the probability of
   a. a fraternal twin's developing a mood disorder given that his or her twin has a mood disorder is approximately 79%.
   *b. an identical twin's developing a mood disorder given that his or her twin has a mood disorder is approximately 79%.
   c. a fraternal twin's developing a mood disorder given that his or her twin has a mood disorder is approximately 48%.
   d. an identical twin's developing a mood disorder given that his or her twin has a mood disorder is approximately 48%.

   Page: 335   Topic: Genetics

48. All of the following have received a great deal of research attention in the hopes of determining what inherited traits make a person susceptible to a mood disorder EXCEPT
   a. faulty neurotransmitter regulation.
   b. faulty hormonal imbalances.
   *c. structural abnormalities in the brain.
   d. disturbances in biological rhythms.

   Page: 335   Topic: What Is Inherited

49. The job of monoamine oxidase (MAO) is to
   a. facilitate the production of neurotransmitters within the vesicles of the synaptic bulb.
   b. regulate the flow of neurotransmitters from axons to dendrites.
   c. inhibit the chemical breakdown and reuptake of neurotransmitters after they have done their job.
   *d. facilitate the chemical breakdown and reuptake of neurotransmitters after they have done their job.

   Page: 336   Topic: Faulty Neurotransmitter Regulation

50. The primary problem with MAO inhibitors is that
   *a. they interact with certain foods to cause such potentially life-threatening conditions as stroke.
   b. their cost is extremely high, making them inaccessible to many people who need them.
   c. prolonged use can lead to irreversible motor problems that cause depressed patients to become more depressed.
   d. they can become addictive.

   Pages: 336–337   Topic: Faulty Neurotransmitter Regulation

51. Menopausal depression, postpartum depression, and premenstrual dysphoric disorder all suggest a connection between mood disorders and
    a. overproduction of neurotransmitters.
    *b. changes in hormone production.
    c. sexual dysfunction.
    d. cyclical changes in levels of serotonin.

    Page: 337   Topic: Faulty Hormonal Regulation

52. The dexamethasone suppression test for determining a hormonal link to depression
    a. shows that depression is caused by high cortisol levels.
    b. shows that depression causes high cortisol levels.
    *c. is not useful because many conditions in addition to depression can affect cortisol regulation.
    d. provides a clear link between hormonal imbalances and the development of mood disorders.

    Page: 337   Topic: Faulty Hormonal Regulation

53. Circadian rhythms reflect
    a. events that occur at night that rely on the gravitational pull of the moon.
    b. seasonal changes that relate to the amount of sunlight in a day.
    c. changes that occur over time from one generation to the next.
    *d. the inner workings of the body's daily biological clock.

    Page: 337   Topic: Biological Rhythms

54. Sleep studies have found that
    *a. partial sleep deprivation may temporarily help depressed people feel better.
    b. allowing depressed people to sleep longer may temporarily help their depression.
    c. depressed people enter REM sleep later in the night than do nondepressed people.
    d. depressed people do not dream as frequently as nondepressed people do.

    Page: 338   Topic: Biological Rhythms

55. According to the psychoanalytic view, depression results from
    a. feelings of worthlessness acquired during toilet training in the anal stage.
    *b. loss of the affection of a parent or another important person during the oral stage.
    c. an inability to establish peer relations during the phallic stage.
    d. child sexual abuse during either the oral or the anal stage.

    Page: 341   Topic: Psychoanalytic Views

56. Dr. Rodriguez believes that mood disorders result from life events that disrupt habitual behaviors. Dr. Rodriguez expresses a _____ view.
    a. psychoanalytic
    b. humanistic
    *c. behavioral
    d. cognitive

    Page: 341   Topic: Behavioral Views

57. All of the following are a part of what Beck calls the cognitive triad of depression EXCEPT
    a. negative feelings about the self.
    b. negative feelings about the world.
    c. negative feelings about the future.
    *d. negative feelings about the past.

    Page: 341   Topic: Cognitive Views

120

58. Angelina is depressed because a young man she has begun dating has not called her in 2 days. She tells her roommate, "I think he has gotten tired of me already." Angelina is demonstrating which logical error?
    *a. arbitrary inference
    b. selected abstraction
    c. overgeneralization
    d. magnification/minimization

    Pages: 341–342   Topic: Cognitive Views

59. According to cognitive psychologists, the four logical errors of thinking stem from
    a. modeling the behavior of others.
    *b. low self-esteem.
    c. being reinforced for demonstrations of humility.
    d. poor cognitive ability.

    Page: 342   Topic: Cognitive Views

60. Rogelio has what Beck would call an autonomous personality. We would expect Rogelio to get his sense of self-esteem from
    a. shows of affection from his family.
    b. support from his friends in time of loss.
    *c. his ability to achieve a desired goal.
    d. acknowledgment by peers of his worthiness.

    Page: 342   Topic: Cognitive Views

61. When an organism, such as a dog or a person, learns that there is no escape from a bad situation and then, when a way out presents itself, makes no effort to escape, the organism's behavior is referred to as
    a. hopelessness.
    b. helplessness.
    c. learned hopelessness.
    *d. learned helplessness.

    Page: 343   Topic: Learned Helplessness

62. People who inherit _____ mood disorders appear to be especially vulnerable to mood swings when faced with stressors.
    *a. a diathesis toward
    b. the gene for
    c. cognitive traits for
    d. their parents'

    Pages: 344–345   Topic: Psychological Diathesis: Current Status

63. The most common biological treatment for mood disorders is
    a. electroconvulsive therapy.
    *b. drug treatment.
    c. light treatment.
    d. sleep deprivation.

    Page: 345   Topic: Biological Treatments

64. Tricyclic antidepressants work by
    a. facilitating the chemical breakdown and reuptake of neurotransmitters after they have done their job.
    b. regulating the flow of neurotransmitters from axons to dendrites.
    *c. blocking the proteins that transport neurotransmitter residues back to synaptic terminals.
    d. increasing the production of the neurotransmitter serotonin.

    Page: 345   Topic: Drug Treatment

65. An important advantage of the selective serotonin reuptake inhibitors such as fluoxetine (Prozac) is that they
    a. work more quickly than other medications.
    b. are more powerful than other medications.
    c. are more effective than other medications.
    *d. have fewer side effects than other medications.

    Page: 346   Topic: Drug Treatment

66. The substance that Australian psychiatrist John Cade accidentally found to treat bipolar disorder, which is now widely used for that disorder, is
    *a. lithium.
    b. imipramine.
    c. fluoxetine.
    d. Prozac.

    Page: 346   Topic: Drug Treatment

67. Electroconvulsive shock therapy (ECT) today differs from its early use in all of the following ways EXCEPT:
    a. patients are given a general anesthetic so they are not conscious during the procedure.
    *b. patients are administered a large dose of insulin instead of electrical current.
    c. patients receive drugs that inhibit body movements.
    d. electrodes are placed only on the right side of the head rather than on both sides.

    Page: 348   Topic: Electroconvulsive Therapy

68. One of the primary problems with the use of ECT is that
    a. it does not work as quickly as some of the newer drugs.
    b. it takes several sessions to bring about any effects.
    *c. memory loss is a side effect of its use.
    d. the treatment does not work well for suicidal patients.

    Page: 348   Topic: Electroconvulsive Therapy

69. Light treatment is most commonly used for
    a. major depressive episodes.
    b. bipolar disorder.
    c. dysthymia.
    *d. seasonal affective disorder.

    Page: 348   Topic: Light Treatment and Sleep Deprivation

70. Interpersonal therapy (IPT) differs from the traditional psychoanalytic approach in all of the following ways EXCEPT:
    *a. IPT helps clients to recognize conflicts such as guilt and self-blame involved in the loss of a loved one.
    b. IPT focuses on the present instead of the past.
    c. IPT clients are taught assertiveness and communication skills.
    d. IPT clients are taught ways to improve their ability to form supportive relationships.

    Page: 349   Topic: Psychoanalytic and Interpersonal Treatment

71. Jeffrey is receiving cognitive-behavioral treatment for his depression. We can expect that in the cognitive component of the treatment Jeffrey will learn to do all of the following EXCEPT
    a. identify self-critical and negative thoughts.
    *b. reinforce himself for positive thoughts.
    c. note the connection between his thoughts and his depression.
    d. challenge negative thoughts to see if they are supportable.

    Page: 349   Topic: Cognitive-Behavioral Treatment

72. Outcome studies have found that
    a. antidepressant medication is the most effective treatment for mood disorders.
    b. cognitive-behavioral treatment and interpersonal treatment are the most effective approaches for curing mood disorders.
    *c. combining psychological treatments with antidepressant medication produces a greater prevention effect than either treatment alone.
    d. so far no therapy has proved itself helpful for mood disorders in the long run.

    Page: 350   Topic: Drugs Versus Psychological Treatment

73. Treatment _____ is measured in the real world, where patients cannot be selected to fit certain profiles and where compliance cannot be guaranteed.
    a. outcome
    b. efficacy
    c. analysis
    *d. effectiveness

    Page: 351   Topic: Critical Thinking About . . . 8.2: Meta-Analysis: Getting the Total Picture

74. Japanese in the 17th century whose failure to their lord was considered a disgrace could expiate themselves only through the suicidal practice of
    *a. Bushido.
    b. hara-kiri.
    c. suttee.
    d. immolation.

    Page: 353   Topic: Suicide

75. While playing Russian roulette—putting one bullet in the chamber of a gun, then twirling the cylinder, holding the gun to his head, and pulling the trigger—Greg fatally shot himself. Although any of the following reasons could explain this suicide, which is the MOST apparent from Greg's actions?
    a. an attempt to extract retribution or obtain martyrdom
    *b. risk taking
    c. mental illness
    d. ending a life of intolerable pain

    Page: 354   Topic: Suicide

76. Suicide rates are related to all of the following EXCEPT
    a. the ambiguity surrounding the death.
    b. social attitudes.
    c. suicide of a celebrity.
    *d. psychological autopsies.

    Page: 354   Topic: Suicide Rates

77. Who is the LEAST likely to attempt suicide?
    *a. Jennifer, an 80-year-old married woman with 10 grandchildren
    b. Harold, an 80-year-old widower with cancer
    c. Ezra, a 65-year-old single man who is an alcoholic
    d. Raul, a 50-year-old divorced man with no family ties

    Page: 355   Topic: Age, Sex, and Ethnic Differences

78. Who is the MOST likely to attempt suicide?
    a. Jeremiah, an African American male
    *b. Washoe, a Native American male
    c. Hiroki, a Japanese American male
    d. Zhao, a Chinese American male

    Page: 355   Topic: Age, Sex, and Ethnic Differences

79. The suicide rate among adolescents has _____ over the past 50 years.
    a. decreased
    b. doubled
    c. tripled
    *d. quadrupled

    Page: 356   Topic: Age, Sex, and Ethnic Differences

80. The typical suicide attempter is
    a. a male adult who shoots himself.
    b. a female adult who slashes her wrists.
    *c. a teenage girl who ingests pills.
    d. an elderly male who hangs himself.

    Page: 357   Topic: Age, Sex, and Ethnic Differences

81. In terms of suicide risk, what time period is the MOST dangerous for someone suffering from a major depressive episode?
    *a. the year following the episode
    b. the month following the episode
    c. in the midst of the episode
    d. the month preceding the episode

    Page: 357   Topic: Psychological Disorders and Suicide

82. According to French sociologist Emile Durkheim, a suicide that results from a person's failure to maintain social ties would be classified as _____ suicide.
    a. an altruistic
    *b. an egoistic
    c. an anomic
    d. a social

    Page: 358   Topic: Sociocultural Factors

83. Especially for adolescents, suicide is associated MOST strongly with
    a. shame and guilt.
    b. anger and revenge.
    *c. hopelessness and impulsivity.
    d. early loss in childhood.

    Page: 359   Topic: Psychological Factors

84. The text states that youthful suicide attempters are alike in
    a. sociocultural background.
    b. having experienced early childhood loss.
    c. feelings of rage.
    *d. lacking problem-solving skills.

    Page: 359   Topic: Psychological Factors

85. Which variables are MOST useful for predicting who will commit suicide?
    *a. early experiences and inherited vulnerabilities that result in a tendency to develop psychological disorders
    b. early experiences of loss that leave a child without the emotional support necessary to develop in a healthy way
    c. inherited vulnerabilities that predispose a person to psychological disorders and suicidal tendencies
    d. an early environment that models and reinforces suicidal behaviors

    Page: 360   Topic: Cause of Suicide: Current Status

86. Which of the following is NOT a high risk factor for suicide?
    a. being male
    *b. living in a rural setting
    c. being single, divorced, or living alone
    d. not regularly attending religious services

    Page: 361   Topic: Table 8.8: Risk Factors and Suicide

87. Ending someone's life to provide a merciful (literally, "good") death is technically referred to as
    a. murder.
    b. assisted suicide.
    *c. euthanasia.
    d. dysthanasia.

    Page: 361   Topic: Treatment and Prevention

88. The first issue to be faced in the treatment of suicide is
    a. finding social support for the patient.
    b. placing the patient in a safe environment.
    c. teaching the patient problem-solving skills.
    *d. assessing the potential for another attempt.

    Page: 361   Topic: Psychological Interventions

89. John F. Kennedy Jr. High School has developed a program to reduce the risk of suicide among its students. One part of the program is a "buddy system" in which students are taught to look out for one another in the hopes that intervention can be started before it is too late. This is a _____ prevention program.
    a. primary
    *b. secondary
    c. tertiary
    d. crisis

    Page: 362   Topic: Primary and Secondary Prevention

90. All of the following are ways to help prevent suicide EXCEPT:
    *a. don't bring up the topic.
    b. regard all threats as serious.
    c. do not keep secrets.
    d. give suicidal people a reason to live.

    Page: 362   Topic: Highlight 8.4: Preventing Suicide: What You Can Do

91. The research by Sloan and colleagues (1990) on restricting guns demonstrated that
    a. strict regulation of the ownership and availability of guns drastically reduced suicides.
    b. strict regulation of the ownership and availability of guns slightly reduced suicides.
    c. despite strict regulation of the ownership and availability of guns, the suicide rate increased.
    *d. despite strict regulation of the ownership and availability of guns, the suicide rate remained unchanged.

    Page: 364   Topic: Reducing Access to Means

92. Postvention, the therapy offered to family and friends of someone who has committed suicide, aims at all of the following EXCEPT
    a. helping relatives and friends cope with grief.
    *b. determining what could have prevented the death.
    c. rumor control.
    d. identifying people at high risk of imitation.

    Page: 364   Topic: Postvention

TRUE-FALSE QUESTIONS

93. A person can be manic or depressed at any given point in time but cannot be both manic and depressed at the same time. (F)

    Page: 318   Topic: Introduction

94. It is not abnormal to feel down after achieving some success. (T)

    Page: 319   Topic: Introduction

95. Mood disorders are exaggerations of everyday emotions. (T)

    Page: 319   Topic: Introduction

96. The mood and the anxiety disorders have been separated in the *DSM* because they are unrelated disorders. (F)

    Page: 322   Topic: Depressive (Unipolar) Disorders

97. It is more likely that physical illness will cause depression than that depression will cause physical illness. (F)

    Pages: 324–325   Topic: Comorbid Conditions

98. The distinction between endogenous and exogenous depression has not proved useful. (T)

    Page: 326   Topic: Major Depressive Disorder

99. Studies using the World Health Organization Depression Screening Instrument have found major national differences in terms of how depression is expressed. (F)

    Page: 328   Topic: Sex, Ethnic, and Cultural Differences

100. In the midst of a manic episode, people find it impossible to focus on a single task. (T)

    Page: 330   Topic: Manic, Hypomanic, and Mixed Episodes

101. People who suffer from mood disorders tend to be more creative than other people. (F)

    Page: 332   Topic: Prevalence and Course of Bipolar Disorders

102. Studies that have found specific genetic markers for mood disorders have been successfully replicated several times. (F)

    Page: 335   Topic: Genetics

103. According to Freud, depression is a form of grief produced in reaction to a loss. (T)

Page: 341   Topic: Psychoanalytic Views

104. The main problem with behavioral explanations of mood disorders is their lack of specificity. (T)

Page: 341   Topic: Behavioral Views

105. Research has demonstrated that depressed people are typically not accurate judges of their own behavior. (F)

Page: 341   Topic: Cognitive Views

106. Mood disorders are less likely among people who have strong social support networks. (T)

Page: 344   Topic: Interpersonal and Social Support

107. Most depressions eventually lift whether they are treated or not. (T)

Page: 346   Topic: Drug Treatment

108. Instead of focusing on the past, interpersonal therapy is concerned with the present. (T)

Page: 349   Topic: Psychoanalytic and Interpersonal Treatment

109. In their comparison of drug therapy with the cognitive-behavioral approach, Rush and colleagues (1977) found drug therapy was superior in the treatment of depression. (F)

Page: 350   Topic: Drugs Versus Psychological Treatment

110. Suicide is influenced by weather. (F)

Page: 353   Topic: Highlight 8.1: Suicide Myths and Reality

111. College students are less likely than non–college students to commit suicide. (F)

Page: 357   Topic: Age, Sex, and Ethnic Differences

112. The overall evidence for the psychoanalytic view of suicide, as a form of murderous anger at another person turned inward against oneself, is not very compelling. (T)

Page: 359   Topic: Psychological Factors

113. The overall evidence indicates that suicide hotlines are highly effective in preventing suicide. (F)

Page: 361   Topic: Crisis Intervention

SHORT-ANSWER QUESTIONS

114. Describe the three stages of grief and how long each lasts.

First comes disbelief, which is replaced within a week or so after the loss with a period of pining for the lost person. In this stage, which may last months or years, people dwell on their loss, have trouble sleeping, neglect other aspects of life, and display anger at their fate. In the final stage, people gradually regain their interest in life, and their sadness abates.

Pages: 320–321   Topic: Grieving

115. Describe the various types of behavior that are typically seen in a major depressive episode.

The hallmark is a sad mood. Depressed people feel down and apathetic. They may go through the motions of daily existence, but there is no enjoyment in it; life seems dull and gray, and formerly pleasurable activities no longer bring enjoyment; starting a new activity seems impossibly difficult; they are constantly tired and just barely drag themselves through life; they may talk and think slowly and may be unable to get out of bed in the morning. However, some depressed people become agitated and are unable to sit still— they pace the floor, shaking their heads, restlessly wringing their hands. Vegetative symptoms include appetite change, sleep disturbance (which may be waking in the night and being unable to get back to sleep, or sleeping constantly), loss of sex drive, and fatigue.

Page: 322   Topic: Major Depressive Episode: Signs

116. Explain the behavioral-relationship cycle that occurs in depression.

Depressed people lose friends and marriage partners because of their pessimism, guilt, and self-blame. They become irritable and short-tempered, snap at their partners and their children, and then, regretting their behavior, feel guilty about mistreating their loved ones. Those feelings of guilt make them even more depressed.

Pages: 322–324   Topic: Major Depressive Episode: Signs

117. According to the text, why do housewives have a higher than average risk of developing depression?

They tend to lose social contacts and feel isolated; they may spend their days brooding about their predicament and yet feel helpless to change their circumstances.

Page: 328   Topic: Sex, Ethnic, and Cultural Differences

118. Describe the characteristics of people experiencing a manic episode.

They find it impossible to focus on a single task, their minds race from one idea to another, they begin various grand projects but do not see them through to completion, their physical activities are energized and chaotic, they have little need for sleep, their sex drive is heightened, they speak quickly and rarely fall silent, their speech is so rapid and they switch topics so often that they may become incoherent.

Pages: 329–330   Topic: Manic, Hypomanic, and Mixed Episodes

119. What are the important diagnostic challenges presented by bipolar disorders, and how are they differentiated from other disorders?

Certain brain tumors may cause manic behaviors, and psychoses can produce a flight from one idea to another. The best way to differentiate bipolar disorder from these other conditions is to focus on mood because few conditions other than bipolar disorder result in an exaggerated elated mood.

Page: 331   Topic: Specific Bipolar Disorders

120. Discuss the different types of studies that are being done to look for a genetic cause of mood disorders; also discuss their findings.

Twin studies compare identical and fraternal twins, who have 100% and approximately 50% of their genes in common, respectively. The concordance rate for identical twins is 70%; for fraternal twins it is around 24%, suggesting that genes play some role in the development of mood disorders. Searches for genetic markers focus on communities that are geographically or socially isolated, in which members either intermarry or have a small number of common ancestors. A study of Orthodox Jewish families in Jerusalem and another with the Amish of Pennsylvania have claimed to find genetic markers, but these studies have not been replicated.

Pages: 334–335   Topic: Genetics

121. What three genetic bases of mood disorders have received the bulk of research attention?

Faulty neurotransmitter regulation, faulty hormonal regulation, and biological rhythms.

Page: 335   Topic: What Is Inherited?

122. Explain the process involved in using the dexamethasone suppression test, and the problems with relying on the results of this test.

When dexamethasone, a synthetic hormone, is taken late in the day, cortisol levels are suppressed throughout the following day in people who are not depressed, but people who are depressed show either no or only minor cortisol suppression the next day, suggesting that depression may be related to some abnormality in the system that regulates cortisol levels. However, it is not clear if depression affects cortisol level, cortisol level affects depression, or some other factor affects both.

Page: 337   Topic: Faulty Hormonal Regulation

123. List the four logical errors proposed by the cognitive view that people with depressive mood disorders use in responding to life events.

arbitrary inference; selected abstraction; overgeneralization; magnification and minimization

Pages: 341–342   Topic: Cognitive Views

124. Differentiate between Beck's notions of sociotropic and autonomous personalities, and state how these personalities relate to depression.

People who are sociotropic value social interaction and intimacy and get their sense of self-esteem from relationships; they would be most likely to develop a mood disorder in response to the loss of a loved one. Those who are autonomous get their sense of self-worth from specific achievements and are most likely to become depressed if they fail to achieve a desired goal.

Page: 342   Topic: Cognitive Views

125. Explain the reasons for, and consequences of, poor patient compliance with use of lithium for bipolar disorder.

Some people stop taking lithium because they like the feeling of well-being and the energy that accompany a manic state; others stop taking it because of the side effects of diarrhea, stomach upset, weakness, and frequent urination. Also, in high doses lithium can be fatal. However, discontinuing lithium increases the probability of a manic episode.

Page: 347   Topic: Drug Treatment

126. What are the basic components of cognitive-behavioral therapy?

In addition to changing thoughts and teaching problem-solving skills, therapists encourage clients to engage in pleasant activities.

Page: 349   Topic: Cognitive-Behavioral Treatment

127. Discuss some of the problems inherent in treatment outcome studies and how these problems are overcome.

Problems include choosing an appropriate dependent measure, selecting treatment and control groups, standardizing treatments, and ensuring that experimenters and subjects are unaware of their status. To judge the effectiveness of a treatment, the results must be synthesized from many different studies, which is done through meta-analysis, a set of techniques designed to find, appraise, and combine data across disparate studies.

Page: 351   Topic: Critical Thinking About . . . 8.2: Meta-Analysis: Getting the Total Picture

128. List the eight suicide myths discussed in the text.

Those who talk about suicide never do it; suicide is related to social class; everyone who commits suicide is depressed; suicide is influenced by the weather ("the suicide season"); suicidal people always want to die; only insane people contemplate suicide; once people try suicide, they remain forever suspect; those who unsuccessfully attempt suicide were never serious.

Page: 353   Topic: Highlight 8.1: Suicide Myths and Reality

ESSAY QUESTIONS

129. Your friend's father died 6 months ago, and your friend still appears to be grieving. Her mother thinks this is abnormal and asks you what is and is not normal. What could you tell her about the wide range of mood disorders, including the various diagnoses; the signs of each; the prevalence and course of each; and the sex, ethnic, and cultural differences among them? Differentiate for your friend's mother the normal from the abnormal characteristics of sadness and grief.

Discuss the various unipolar and bipolar disorders and how they can be differentiated from normal behavior.

130. After many years of being apart, you finally reconnect with an old friend who had moved away during grade school. He tells you he has had a difficult time these past several years—and that he spent 2 years in a mental health facility and was just released a month ago. Despite his many bouts with depression and his cousin's bouts with bipolar disorder (which ultimately ended in her suicide), your friend tells you he really doesn't understand what causes the mood disorders. What could you tell him about the etiology of the mood disorders?

Discuss the genetics of mood disorders including what is inherited, and the psychosocial factors involved, including the various views about etiology.

131. One of your neighbors confides in you that her son has bipolar disorder and her daughter has just been diagnosed with seasonal affective disorder. Your neighbor is concerned about the treatments that her children are undergoing, and she also tells you about the treatment she received for depression shortly after she was married. She wants to know if she was given the "right" treatment and what kinds of treatment would be appropriate for her children. She wonders if perhaps no treatment at all would be better. What could you tell her about the various types of treatment for the mood disorders?

Address the biological treatments and the psychological treatments, indicating which type of treatment is typically used in the different disorders; then address the problem of undertreatment.

132. A local therapist has just been invited to campus to talk to students about a student's recent suicide. Your friends are talking about this in the cafeteria, and they ask you about the relationship between mood disorders and suicide. One of them believes that if someone wants to die, he or she should be allowed to do it. Another is horrified at that opinion and wants to know exactly who is at risk and what the causes of suicide are. What could you tell your friends about these issues?

Discuss what suicide is; its prevalence, incidence, and risk factors; and the various causes of suicide.

133. Lately it seems there has been an increase in suicides at the local high schools and colleges, and many students who aren't attempting suicide are nonetheless experiencing major depressive episodes. Knowing of your interest in this area, a community leader approaches you to ask for your help in designing a suicide prevention program that would help young people deal with (or avoid) mood disorders, as well as try to prevent suicide and help survivors deal with the suicides of their loved ones. Describe all the issues you would need to address, and outline a program that you think would help.

Discuss how to assess suicidal intentions. Then evaluate the various types of treatment and prevention, including crisis intervention, psychological interventions, primary and secondary prevention, reducing access to means, and postvention.

CHAPTER 9
THE SCHIZOPHRENIAS AND
OTHER PSYCHOTIC DISORDERS

MULTIPLE-CHOICE QUESTIONS

1. The most catastrophic of all psychological disorders is
    *a. schizophrenia.
    b. antisocial personality disorder.
    c. depression.
    d. bipolar disorder.

    Page: 370   Topic: Introduction

2. Which of the following is NOT a reason that schizophrenia presents major problems to those who suffer from it, as well as to their families and society at large?
    a. Schizophrenia wrecks the social relationships and impairs the thinking of those who suffer from it, and it robs them of the ability to enjoy life.
    *b. The high cost of dealing with schizophrenia arises from costs of hospitalization and the dangers that schizophrenics pose to society.
    c. Few people with schizophrenia can work, many require public assistance, and most need expensive treatment.
    d. Faced with unrewarding lives, people with schizophrenia may commit suicide, adding yet another burden to the guilt and pain their families already bear.

    Page: 370   Topic: Introduction

3. A critical way in which schizophrenia differs from most other psychological disorders is that
    a. schizophrenia is a more severe disorder.
    b. the onset of schizophrenia is much earlier than the onset of most other disorders.
    *c. people with schizophrenia behave in ways that most other people find incomprehensible.
    d. people with schizophrenia exhibit more dangerous behavior than people with other disorders do.

    Page: 372   Topic: The Genesis of Schizophrenia

4. Disorders characterized by gross distortions of reality are called
    a. neuroses.
    b. pareses.
    c. psychopathologies.
    *d. psychoses.

    Page: 372   Topic: The Genesis of Schizophrenia

5. One of the first people to advocate separating and classifying disorders according to their main features was
    *a. Phillipe Pinel.
    b. Benedict Morel.
    c. Emil Kraepelin.
    d. Eugen Bleuler.

    Page: 372   Topic: The Genesis of Schizophrenia

6.Pinel believed it was important to classify psychological disorders according to their main features so that they could be
   a. properly treated.
   *b. traced back to their physiological causes.
   c. diagnosed according to their severity.
   d. better understood.

   Page: 372   Topic: The Genesis of Schizophrenia

7. Emil Kraepelin used the term *dementia praecox* to refer to
   a. symptoms that follow a cyclical course in which periods of remission alternate with psychotic episodes.
   b. deterioration of the brain that results in loss of memory, irrational behavior, and ultimately death.
   *c. serious mental symptoms that begin early in life and follow a deteriorating course.
   d. serious mental symptoms that may begin at any point in life and follow a deteriorating course.

   Page: 372   Topic: The Genesis of Schizophrenia

8. When proposing that the term *schizophrenia* replace the term *dementia praecox,* Bleuler used the former term to describe
   a. the splitting of an individual's personality.
   b. an alternation of extreme euphoria and deep depression.
   c. a split from reality.
   *d. a disconnecting of a person's thoughts from each other.

   Page: 373   Topic: The Genesis of Schizophrenia

9. Which of the following is a symptom that Bleuler would classify as "accessory"?
   *a. hallucinations
   b. loss of initiative
   c. impaired attention
   d. ambivalence

   Page: 374   Topic: The Genesis of Schizophrenia

10. Delusions are
   a. sensory experiences in the absence of external stimuli.
   *b. unsubstantiated beliefs.
   c. odd motor movements.
   d. bizarre behaviors.

   Page: 374   Topic: The Genesis of Schizophrenia

11. Kurt Schneider's (1959) classification of first-rank symptoms (hearing one's own voice being spoken aloud, hearing voices commenting on one's own behavior, and the feeling that one's actions are controlled by other people) has been
   a. substantiated by mental health professionals today as being specific to schizophrenia.
   b. shown by mental health professionals today not to be indicative of schizophrenia.
   *c. designated as indicative of schizophrenia, as well as of other disorders.
   d. shown by mental health professionals to represent exaggerations of normal behaviors.

   Page: 374   Topic: The Genesis of Schizophrenia

12. Compared with their European counterparts, American mental health workers in the 1970s were _____ likely to diagnose a patient as schizophrenic.
    a. equally as
    b. half as
    c. slightly less
    *d. twice as

    Page: 374   Topic: The Genesis of Schizophrenia

13. Dr. Schmitz was a psychologist in Germany, but she has now moved to California and has recently passed the state exams so that she can practice in that state as a clinical psychologist. We would expect that the criteria she employed in her European diagnostic experience
    *a. would have been quite similar to the diagnostic criteria used in the United States.
    b. would have been similar to those used in the United States for severe disorders such as schizophrenia, but would have differed for the less severe disorders.
    c. would have been dissimilar to the diagnostic criteria used in the United States.
    d. would reflect cultural differences.

    Page: 374   Topic: The Genesis of Schizophrenia

14. If Bleuler was correct, then
    a. schizophrenia is the same as a "split personality."
    *b. schizophrenia is not a single disorder.
    c. there may be a single underlying cause for schizophrenia.
    d. environmental factors may change the way schizophrenia is manifested.

    Page: 374   Topic: Symptoms and Signs

15. Gerald has symptoms that are similar to those of schizophrenia, but his symptoms have not yet become chronic. Gerald would be diagnosed with
    a. schizoaffective disorder.
    b. shared psychotic disorder.
    *c. schizophreniform disorder.
    d. brief psychotic disorder.

    Page: 374   Topic: Symptoms and Signs

16. _____ disorder is a combination of schizophrenic symptoms and mood disorder.
    a. Schizophreniform
    b. Delusional
    c. Shared psychotic
    *d. Schizoaffective

    Page: 375   Topic: Symptoms and Signs

17. Mildred and her 25-year-old daughter, Mollie, have lived together since Mollie was widowed two years ago. They both believe that their thoughts are being monitored by the government and that Mollie's deceased husband plans to murder them. Mildred and Mollie would most likely be diagnosed as having
    *a. shared psychotic disorder.
    b. schizophrenia.
    c. schizoaffective disorder.
    d. delusional disorder.

    Page: 375   Topic: Symptoms and Signs

18. All of the following are characteristic symptoms of schizophrenia listed in *DSM-IV* EXCEPT
    a. delusions.
    *b. social dysfunction.
    c. hallucinations.
    d. disorganized speech.

    Page: 375   Topic: Table 9.1: Main *DSM-IV* Psychotic Disorders

19. Which of the following is a positive symptom of schizophrenia?
    a. loss of initiative
    b. lack of emotional expression
    *c. bizarre motor movements
    d. impoverished speech

    Page: 375   Topic: Positive versus Negative Symptoms

20. To be considered a potential symptom of schizophrenia, delusions must be
    a. unsubstantiated.
    b. visual.
    c. out of touch with reality.
    *d. contrary to a person's background.

    Page: 376   Topic: Delusions

21. When a person produces little speech, and the speech that is produced is slow and devoid of content, this is referred to as
    *a. alogia.
    b. aphasia.
    c. atoxia.
    d. mutism.

    Page: 376   Topic: Delusions

22. The text notes that delusions may serve what purpose?
    a. They frighten other people away, which may provide people with schizophrenia some degree of comfort by keeping them socially isolated.
    *b. They may help to protect people with schizophrenia from having to admit to themselves that their experiences and behaviors result from a mental disorder.
    c. They provide a pathway of clues that would allow someone who truly cares to reach someone with schizophrenia.
    d. They are a way for people with schizophrenia to organize their disordered world.

    Pages: 376–377   Topic: Delusions

23. _____ delusions have the greatest diagnostic value.
    a. Plausible
    b. Vague
    *c. Bizarre
    d. Systematic

    Page: 377   Topic: Delusions

24. Frank has Capgras's syndrome. He believes that
    a. the government is monitoring his thoughts.
    b. the government is trying to insert thoughts into his mind.
    c. he is dead.
    *d. his parents have been replaced by doubles.

    Page: 377   Topic: Delusions

25. Perceptions that occur without any external stimulus are referred to as
    *a. hallucinations.
    b. delusions.
    c. misperceptions.
    d. negative symptoms.

    Page: 377   Topic: Hallucinations

26. The most common type of hallucinations are
    a. visual.
    *b. auditory.
    c. olfactory.
    d. tactile.

    Page: 377   Topic: Hallucinations

27. Using the technique of cerebral blood flow monitoring, researchers have found that the area of the brain that is most active during a patient's auditory hallucinations is the area responsible for
    a. language comprehension.
    b. visual processing.
    *c. speech production.
    d. auditory processing.

    Page: 378   Topic: Hallucinations

28. Jennifer Plowman (the case study in the chapter) exhibited many examples of disorganized speech. For example, she jumped from one topic to another in a seemingly unrelated way. This type of disorganized speech is referred to as
    a. neologisms.
    b. clanging.
    c. word salad.
    *d. thought derailment.

    Page: 378   Topic: Disorganized Speech

29. Catherine has remained in the same position, without moving, for 3 hours. Another patient walks by her and moves Catherine's arms out to the side, and they remain there until an orderly comes by and moves them down to their normal position. This demonstrates a catatonic symptom called
    *a. waxy flexibility.
    b. autism.
    c. excitement.
    d. encephalitis lethargica.

    Page: 378   Topic: Disorganized or Catatonic Behavior

30. In the case study in the text, Jennifer Plowman's facial expression is described as being devoid of emotion. Such an expression is referred to as
    a. inappropriate affect.
    *b. flat affect.
    c. anhedonia.
    d. positive affect.

    Page: 379   Topic: Flat or Inappropriate Affect

31. If Eduardo is suffering from schizophrenia and exhibits flat affect, it is likely that he
    a. is experiencing little or no emotion.
    b. does not know how to express his emotions.
    *c. is experiencing emotions, but does not show his feelings.
    d. has been taught to keep his feelings to himself.

    Page: 379   Topic: Flat or Inappropriate Affect

32. Erica, who is being treated for schizophrenia, has withdrawn from everyday social interaction and has retreated into her own personal fantasy world. As noted in the text, she has probably done this for all of the following reasons EXCEPT that she
    a. needs to minimize her sensory stimulation.
    b. feels a need to protect herself from further loss of control.
    c. does not have the energy she needs to keep up with everyday activities.
    *d. believes it is the best way to gain control of her life.

    Page: 379   Topic: Social Withdrawal and Lethargy

33. For a diagnosis of schizophrenia, all of the following must be ruled out EXCEPT
    *a. prodromal phases.
    b. mood disorders.
    c. pervasive developmental disorders.
    d. substance abuse.

    Page: 379   Topic: Additional Symptoms and Signs

34. Xavier has been diagnosed with schizophrenia. From his frozen body posture, or stupor, we can tell that his subtype is
    a. paranoid.
    *b. catatonic.
    c. disorganized.
    d. hebephrenic.

    Page: 380   Topic: Diagnostic Issues: Subtypes

35. Based on Jennifer Plowman's symptoms of vague, incoherent delusions, incoherent speech, and flat affect, in the case study in our text, Dr. Kahn has assigned Jennifer to which subtype of schizophrenia?
    a. paranoid
    b. catatonic
    *c. disorganized
    d. undifferentiated

    Page: 380   Topic: Diagnostic Issues

36. Those who object to the diagnosis of schizophrenia, such as Thomas Szasz (1961, 1971), have done so for all of the following reasons EXCEPT:
    a. there is no "gold standard" by which the accuracy of the diagnosis of schizophrenia can be judged.
    b. the population of people with schizophrenia is so heterogeneous, it is difficult to say they all have the same disorder.
    c. clinicians do not always agree with each other when making a diagnosis.
    *d. schizophrenia appears to be culture specific, and thus may be an artifact of how Western clinicians diagnose individuals with these symptoms.

    Page: 381   Topic: Objections to the Diagnosis of Schizophrenia

37. Most typically, schizophrenia makes its first appearance in
    *a. adolescence.
    b. early adulthood.
    c. middle adulthood.
    d. childhood.

    Page: 382   Topic: Course of Schizophrenia

38. The phase that precedes active schizophrenia is referred to as the _____ phase.
    a. residual
    *b. prodromal
    c. preparatory
    d. stability

    Page: 382   Topic: Prodromal Phase

39. To keep from disintegrating further, individuals in the prodromal phase of schizophrenia may
    a. seek help from a therapist.
    b. engage in greater social contact to slow the progression of the disorder.
    *c. consciously try to control their thoughts and actions.
    d. engage in ritualistic behaviors.

    Pages: 382–383   Topic: Prodromal Phase

40. Which of the following patients is most likely to have a successful recovery from schizophrenia?
    a. Angela, whose delusions and speech are difficult to understand
    b. Brenda, who has incoherent speech and flat affect
    c. Carol, who is catatonic, extremely negative, and socially withdrawn
    *d. Deborah, who believes she is the Archangel Gabriel and communicates with God

    Page: 384   Topic: Residual Phase

41. The relapse rate for people with schizophrenia is worst for those whose first episode occurred
    *a. when they were children.
    b. in adolescence.
    c. in early adulthood.
    d. later in life.

    Page: 384   Topic: Residual Phase

42. The number of new cases that appears during a period of time is referred to as the _____
    of a disorder.
    a. prevalence
    *b. incidence
    c. rate
    d. epidemiology

    Page: 385   Topic: Incidence

43. Epidemiological studies of schizophrenia around the world indicate that
    a. rates are higher in industrialized nations than in nonindustrialized nations.
    b. rates are higher in nonindustrialized nations than in industrialized nations.
    *c. rates are remarkably similar around the world.
    d. current methods of data collection make it difficult to determine if rates are similar around the world.

    Page: 385   Topic: Incidence

44. Which type of schizophrenia appears to have become less common in industrialized nations?
    a. paranoid
    b. disorganized
    c. undifferentiated
    *d. catatonic

    Page: 386   Topic: Incidence

45. Cross-culturally, it has been noted that the age of onset for schizophrenia
    *a. is earlier for males than for females.
    b. is earlier for females than for males.
    c. is the same for both males and females.
    d. depends on the particular culture.

    Page: 386   Topic: Age of Onset

46. Who has the worst prognosis in terms of chronicity and seriousness of schizophrenia?
    a. Janine, a 30-year-old female who was diagnosed after the death of her husband last year
    *b. Ken, a 19-year-old male who began to show prodromal symptoms in mid-adolescence
    c. Luther, a 50-year-old male who was hospitalized for the first time a month ago
    d. Marny, a 22-year-old female who was first diagnosed by Student Health Services after her sophomore year of college

    Page: 387   Topic: Age of Onset

47. Dr. Rosen is studying the number of cases of schizophrenia at a given time. She is looking specifically at
    a. period prevalence.
    b. lifetime prevalence.
    *c. point prevalence.
    d. overall prevalence.

    Page: 387   Topic: Prevalence

48. The reason stated in the text for a higher prevalence of schizophrenia in certain areas is
    a. politics.
    b. culture.
    c. religious practices.
    *d. migration.

    Page: 387   Topic: Prevalence

49. A critical factor that needs to be accounted for when comparing prevalence rates of schizophrenia cross-culturally is
    *a. age.
    b. time of study.
    c. economic differences.
    d. gender.

    Page: 386   Topic: Critical Thinking About . . . 9.1: Standardizing Across Cultures

50. Which of the following statements is NOT a problem with Gottesman's (1991) findings of the genetic heritability of schizophrenia?
    a. Sixty-three percent of schizophrenic probands in the studies Gottesman analyzed did not have any relatives with schizophrenia.
    *b. The connection in the Danish high-risk study was between schizophrenia and schizotypal personality traits.
    c. In the studies that Gottesman analyzed, it was often difficult to determine if the twins were monozygotic or dizygotic.
    d. The studies Gottesman analyzed differed in terms of sampling biases, diagnostic criteria, and other methodological problems.

    Pages: 388–389   Topic: Family Studies

51. The strongest confirmation that Gottesman and his colleagues found in their twin studies to support a genetic basis for schizophrenia was that
    a. monozygotic twins have much higher concordance rates for schizophrenia than do dizygotic twins.
    b. the degree of blood relationship correlates strongly with rates of schizophrenia.
    *c. the probability of a child's developing schizophrenia is 17% whether it is the child's parent or the parent's identical twin who is schizophrenic.
    d. events that occur in the intrauterine environment during pregnancy were not found to affect whether a child would later become schizophrenic.

    Page: 391   Topic: Twin Studies

52. Aisha was adopted when she was 1 week old. Her biological mother is schizophrenic, but her adoptive parents are mentally healthy. In terms of her risk for developing schizophrenia, Aisha is
    a. less likely to develop schizophrenia than she would be if she were being raised by her biological mother.
    b. more likely to develop schizophrenia than she would be if she were being raised by her biological mother.
    c. likely to develop schizophrenia only if she experiences a major trauma in her life.
    *d. no more likely to develop schizophrenia than she would be if she were being raised by her biological mother.

    Page: 392   Topic: Adoption Studies

53. Zander has been diagnosed with schizophrenia, and, as might be expected in terms of his cognitive functioning, he did not perform well on the Continuous Performance Test (CPT), which required him to identify a target letter in a rapidly presented display of letters. With respect to his relatives, we would expect to see that
    *a. Zander's relatives who are not schizophrenic would also have difficulty with the CPT.
    b. Zander's relatives who are not schizophrenic would have little, if any, difficulty with the CPT.
    c. Zander's parents and siblings would have difficulty with the CPT, but other relatives would not.
    d. only Zander's siblings would have difficulty with the CPT.

    Page: 393   Topic: Attentional Dysfunction

54. Which of the following is NOT a reason for believing that schizophrenia is polygenic?
    a. Polygenic inheritance would explain why only 17% of the offspring of a parent with schizophrenia develop the condition themselves.
    *b. An individual may carry the genotype for schizophrenia but display varying degrees of psychopathology.
    c. Polygenic inheritance may account for schizophrenia's varied course and symptoms.
    d. When several genes are responsible for a condition, a single genetic marker would not be present in all cases.

    Page: 394   Topic: How Many Genes Are Involved in Schizophrenia?

55. According to the diathesis-stress model, the symptoms of schizophrenia are most likely
    a. inherited.
    b. the result of environmental influences.
    *c. the result of an interaction between genetic and nongenetic factors.
    d. to be exhibited if a person's identical twin is schizophrenic.

    Page: 395   Topic: How Many Genes Are Involved in Schizophrenia?

56. Researchers who are examining season of birth are typically looking at which risk factor for schizophrenia?
    a. life-stress
    b. social class
    c. brain chemistry
    *d. viral infection

    Page: 395   Topic: Viral Infection

57. In the search for nongenetic risk factors for schizophrenia, a particularly important variable that has found much support in the research is
    *a. social class.
    b. life-stress.
    c. season of birth.
    d. homelessness.

    Page: 397   Topic: Demographic and Socioeconomic Status

58. Due to his schizophrenia, Glen is impaired in his ability to hold a job. As a result, when not living on the streets, he lives in a poor neighborhood. His father, an artist, and his mother, a college professor, live in an upscale section of the same city. This demonstrates which theory?
    a. social stress theory
    *b. social drift theory
    c. neurodevelopmental theory
    d. life-stress theory

    Page: 397   Topic: Demographic and Socioeconomic Status

59. Which of the following has been linked to return to the hospital or exacerbation of symptoms for patients with schizophrenia?
    a. a schizophrenogenic mother
    b. low communication
    *c. expressed emotion
    d. direct communication

    Page: 398   Topic: Communication and Expressed Emotion

60. The most commonly reported brain abnormality among those with schizophrenia is
    a. smaller brain density.
    b. increased activity in the frontal lobe.
    c. larger hippocampus and amygdala.
    *d. larger ventricles.

    Page: 399   Topic: Brain Structure and Function

61. The neurotransmitter that has received the most focus in research into the relationship between brain chemistry and schizophrenia is
   *a. dopamine.
   b. serotonin.
   c. glutamate.
   d. ACTH.

   Page: 401   Topic: Brain Chemistry

62. A major problem with the hypothesis that schizophrenic symptoms result from excessive dopamine activity comes from research with
   a. the drug L-dopa.
   *b. LSD and PCP.
   c. antipsychotic medications.
   d. phenothiazines.

   Page: 401   Topic: Brain Chemistry

63. Dr. Stolz is investigating the hypothesis that excess dopamine receptors are a causative factor in schizophrenia. A problem with this research would be that
   a. the participants in the studies all have schizophrenia, so it is unknown whether there are people without schizophrenia who also have excess dopamine receptors.
   b. people with schizophrenia who have excess dopamine receptors also have more receptors for many other neurotransmitters.
   *c. most people with schizophrenia receive drug treatment, which may be the cause of the extra dopamine receptors.
   d. while increasing dopamine receptors, drug therapy for schizophrenia decreases serotonin receptors; that may be the cause of the symptoms.

   Page: 401   Topic: Brain Chemistry

64. If Sara is receiving milieu treatment, we would most likely find her
   a. in a halfway house.
   b. living in her own community.
   c. in group therapy.
   *d. in a hospital environment.

   Page: 403   Topic: Hospitalization and Milieu Treatment

65. The precursor to modern civil commitment laws was
   *a. the vagrancy act passed by the British Parliament to detain the "furiously mad."
   b. the restraining of mental patients in chains in London's St. Mary of Bethlehem Hospital.
   c. moral-religious treatment of the mentally ill in William Tuke's York Retreat.
   d. the squalid living conditions of 18th-century England that drove people mad.

   Page: 403   Topic: From Community to Asylum and Back Again

66. Antipsychotic medications developed in the 1960s made it possible for people with mental disorders to live outside the hospital environment. Patients were discharged in a process known as
   a. back to the community.
   *b. deinstitutionalization.
   c. moral treatment.
   d. decommitment.

   Page: 405   Topic: From Community to Asylum and Back Again

67. Nancy was hospitalized against her will under the civil commitment laws. She has all of the following rights EXCEPT
    a.   the right to receive or to refuse treatment.
    b.   the right to be housed in humane conditions.
    *c. the right to be treated on an outpatient basis.
    d.   the right to know the consequences of a treatment.

    Page: 404   Topic: Highlight 9.l: Civil Commitment

68. The aim of deinstitutionalization was that mental patients be helped within their communities rather than institutionalized in hospitals. What appears to have been the outcome of that movement?
    a.   For the most part, communities have provided excellent support and resources for the mentally ill.
    b.   Although not as many community facilities have been funded to help the mentally ill as envisioned, for the most part halfway houses have filled the gap.
    c.   Due to the lack of service provision in the community, the mentally ill are now returning to the mental hospitals.
    *d. The situation is grossly inequitable in that the wealthy find their way into private hospitals and the poor often wind up on the streets.

    Page: 406   Topic: Deinstitutionalization

69. Which statement about neuroleptics is FALSE?
    *a. They are equally as effective for reducing the positive and the negative symptoms of schizophrenia.
    b.   They are equally as effective for people from different racial backgrounds.
    c.   They are not effective for approximately 25% of those with schizophrenia.
    d.   They present a risk of side effects, such as a shuffling walk, shakiness, and other odd movements.

    Page: 407   Topic: Somatic Treatments

70. Amalia, who has been hospitalized for her schizophrenia, is now being released. The therapeutic team working on Amalia's case decided that the best approach for her recovery is to reduce expressed emotion. Therefore, we would expect that
    a.   Amalia would be trained to monitor her emotions so she is careful to avoid explosive episodes.
    *b. among other things, her family would be taught to lower their level of expressed emotion.
    c.   Amalia would be trained in ways to lower her levels of expressed emotion.
    d.   the therapeutic team would express lower levels of emotion with Amalia when her behavior is inappropriate.

    Page: 409   Topic: Reducing Expressed Emotion

71. Token economies are based on the principles of
    a.   social learning theory.
    b.   classical conditioning.
    *c. operant conditioning.
    d.   aversive conditioning.

    Page: 410   Topic: Token Economies

72. Hector is receiving social skills training to help him learn the basics of social interaction. With respect to this specific type of training, Hector will be involved in all of the following EXCEPT
    a.   role playing.
    b.   modeling.
    c.   programmed learning techniques.
    *d. examining his thoughts.

    Page: 410   Topic: Social Skills and Cognitive Training

TRUE-FALSE QUESTIONS

73. Schizophrenia is a specific disorder characterized by severe psychological symptoms. (F)
    Page: 368   Topic: Chapter Objectives

74. The modern schizophrenic syndrome originated in the 18th century. (T)
    Page: 372   Topic: The Genesis of Schizophrenia

75. The basic underlying symptom of schizophrenia is bizarre thoughts. (F)
    Page: 375   Topic: Symptoms and Signs

76. Because the only difference between schizophreniform disorder and schizophrenia is the duration of symptoms, schizophreniform disorder should be considered a provisional diagnosis. (T)
    Page: 375   Topic: Symptoms and Signs

77. People with delusional disorder meet most, but not all, of the criteria for schizophrenia. (F)
    Page: 375   Topic: Symptoms and Signs

78. A diagnosis of schizophrenia involves social and/or occupational dysfunction. (T)
    Page: 375   Topic: Symptoms and Signs

79. A diagnosis of schizophrenia can be made only after other alternatives (e.g., substance abuse) are excluded. (T)
    Page: 376   Topic: Symptoms and Signs/Table 9.2: Main *DSM-IV* Diagnosic Criteria for Schizophrenia

80. Delusions are most typically vague and incoherent. (F)
    Page: 377   Topic: Delusions

81. A person who has delusions may otherwise be perfectly rational. (T)
    Page: 377   Topic: Delusions

82. The most common type of hallucinations are visual. (F)
    Page: 377   Topic: Hallucinations

83. The part of the brain that is most active during schizophrenic auditory hallucinations is in the area responsible for speech production. (T)
    Page: 378   Topic: Hallucinations

84. Disorganized speech may be found in both schizophrenia and bipolar disorder. (T)
    Page: 378   Topic: Disorganized Speech

85. Most people with schizophrenia speak quite differently from people who do not have the disorder. (F)
    Page: 378   Topic: Disorganized Speech

86. Children who later develop schizophrenia typically are less emotionally responsive and have poorer motor coordination than their siblings who do not develop the disorder. (T)
    Page: 379   Topic: Flat or Inappropriate Affect

87. The subtype classifications of schizophrenia are helpful to clinicians in predicting who will respond to treatment. (F)

    Page: 380   Topic: Diagnostic Issues: Subtypes

88. Overall, outcomes for people with schizophrenia are better in developing countries than in the developed world. (T)

    Page: 384   Topic: Residual Phase

89. Good premorbid adjustment, acute onset, and the absence of neurological abnormalities predict recovery in schizophrenia. (F)

    Page: 384   Topic: Process Versus Reactive Schizophrenia

90. Schizophrenia has remained recognizable in all times and in industrial and nonindustrial societies around the world. (T)

    Page: 385   Topic: Incidence, Age of Onset, and Prevalence

91. Being raised by a parent with schizophrenia makes a child more likely to develop schizophrenia. (F)

    Page: 392   Topic: Adoption Studies

92. There is no cure for schizophrenia. (T)

    Page: 402   Topic: Treatment

SHORT-ANSWER QUESTIONS

93. What is it about schizophrenia that makes it the "most catastrophic of all psychological disorders"?

    It typically strikes young adults, who may suffer for decades; it wrecks social relationships, impairs thinking, and robs those who have it of the ability to enjoy life; because few schizophrenics are able to work, many require public assistance; most require expensive treatment; many commit suicide, causing even more guilt and pain for their friends and families.

    Page: 370   Topic: Introduction

94. How do delusions differ from hallucinations?

    Delusions are unsubstantiated beliefs; hallucinations are sensory experiences in the absence of external stimuli.

    Page: 374   Topic: The Genesis of Schizophrenia

95. How do schizophreniform disorder and schizoaffective disorder differ from schizophrenia?

    Schizophreniform disorder has not yet become chronic; schizoaffective disorder is a combination of symptoms of schizophrenia and mood disorder, but the delusions and hallucinations must be present for at least 2 weeks in the absence of any mood symptoms.

    Pages: 374–375   Topic: Symptoms and Signs

96. Differentiate between the positive and the negative symptoms of schizophrenia.

    Positive symptoms reflect an excess or distortion of normal cognitive and emotional functions (e.g., delusions, hallucinations, bizarre motor movements); negative symptoms reflect a reduction or loss of normal functions (e.g., loss of initiative, lack of emotional expression, impoverished speech).

    Page: 375   Topic: Positive Versus Negative Symptoms

97. Describe the different types of disorganized speech that are characteristic of schizophrenia.

    Neologisms: made-up words, such as Jennifer Plowman's "logomouth" and "selegonit." Derailment: jumping from one topic to the next. Clang associations: linking words together according to their sound (come, lum, rum). Tangentiality: irrelevant responses to questions. Word salad: a mass of disconnected words.

    Page: 378   Topic: Disorganized Speech

98. Differentiate among the different subtypes of schizophrenia.

    Paranoid: delusions or auditory hallucinations without disorganized speech, catatonic behavior, or flat or inappropriate affect. Disorganized: incoherent speech accompanied by bizarre and sometimes childish behavior, plus flat or inappropriate affect. Catatonic: odd motor activity (e.g., immobility, waxy flexibility, excessive motor activity, etc.). Undifferentiated: when someone meets the diagnostic criteria but does not fit a specific subtype. Residual: negative symptoms or mild versions of positive symptoms.

    Page: 380   Topic: Diagnostic Issues: Subtypes

99. What are the primary objections to the diagnosis of schizophrenia?

    There is no "gold standard" for making an accurate diagnosis; because schizophrenia is a heterogeneous syndrome and its diagnosis requires that only two of five possible symptoms be present, with no one symptom receiving greater weight than any other, the diagnosis can be applied to very different people; clinicians do not always agree when making the diagnosis; and some writers believe that schizophrenia is not a mental disorder, but a moral judgment made by the middle-class majority about the odd behavior of an eccentric minority.

    Page: 381   Topic: Objections to the Diagnosis of Schizophrenia

100. Describe the three phases of schizophrenia.

    Prodromal phase: precedes the disorder and is marked by a deterioration from a higher level of functioning, typically with negative symptoms appearing before positive symptoms. Active phase: patients no longer seem to be aware that they are behaving strangely and show full-blown symptoms. Residual phase: negative symptoms and mild levels of positive symptoms persist after the passing of the active phase. In "single" episodes, the active phase is followed by a period in which there are either no symptoms or only negative ones.

    Pages: 382–383   Topic: Course of Schizophrenia

101. Explain why there appears to be a more positive course for schizophrenia in developing nations.

    First, the more positive result may be artifactual: societies that are more accepting of divergent behavior may rate an outcome as more favorable even if it is identical to an outcome not deemed favorable in a developed country. Alternatively, something in the social environment of developing countries may produce a more positive outcome.

    Pages: 384–385   Topic: Course and Culture

102. What problems arise from determining incidence estimates for schizophrenia by counting the number of new cases seen at treatment facilities over a 1-year period?

    It makes two untrue assumptions: first, that all cases are seen at such treatment facilities and second, that clinicians who work at them are perfectly accurate in their diagnoses.

    Pages: 385–386   Topic: Incidence

103. Describe the types of studies that have been used to understand the genetic bases of schizophrenia.

Family studies: after a patient (the proband) is identified, the proband's relatives are examined to see whether any suffer from schizophrenia or another psychotic disorder. Twin studies: the incidence of schizophrenia in monozygotic and dizygotic twins is examined; if genetic factors determine who develops schizophrenia, monozygotic twins reared together would be expected to show a higher rate of concordance for schizophrenia than would dizygotic twins reared together. Adoption studies: after identifying schizophrenic probands adopted soon after birth, the psychological histories of each proband's natural and adoptive families are investigated for psychotic disorders. Markers: after cognitive markers for attentional dysfunction and eye-tracking abnormalities are identified, persons with those markers are followed to see if they develop schizophrenia.

Pages: 387–394   Topic: Etiology of Schizophrenia: Genetics

104. What nongenetic risk factors for schizophrenia does the text suggest have found some support?

viral infection; life-stress; social class; low socioeconomic status; expressed emotion; brain structure and function; brain chemistry

Page: 395   Topic: Etiology of Schizophrenia: Nongenetic Risk Factors

105. Explain the two general ideas driving deinstitutionalization.

Deinstitutionalization is based on the belief that mental patients are better cared for in their home communities, where they are known and where they can participate in everyday life, and on the notion that mental hospitals are repressive environments that do more harm than good and that patients should be provided with the least restrictive environment possible.

Pages: 405 and 407   Topic: Deinstitutionalization

106. What are the most serious side effects of neuroleptic medications?

In addition to a shuffling walk, expressionless face, shakiness, and odd movements, the most serious is the generally irreversible iatrogenic movement disorder known as tardive dyskinesia. Symptoms include facial grimaces, jerky movements, lip chewing, and other tics and movements.

Page: 407   Topic: Somatic Treatments

107. Describe the psychological treatments for schizophrenia that were discussed in the text.

Reducing expressed emotion: the education of families about the types of behavior to expect of the patient, the provision of information about medications, including their side effects and monitoring of their use, and the provision of training in problem-solving and communication skills. Token economies: elaborate reinforcement programs in which desired behaviors are rewarded with a token that can be exchanged for privileges. Social skills: the teaching of skills such as how to interview for a job, hold a conversation, etc. Cognitive behavior therapy: the provision of education about schizophrenia and how to monitor one's own behavior.

Pages: 409–410   Topic: Psychological Treatment

ESSAY QUESTIONS

108. Your roommate's brother knows you are taking this class in abnormal psychology, so he approaches you in confidence. He says that lately he has noticed his favorite cousin has been acting strangely. He tells you that the cousin has been saying they must whisper all their conversations because everything she thinks and says is being monitored by the government. When not focused on that concern, she seems to be able to carry on a somewhat coherent conversation, but he has also noticed that her hygiene seems to be slipping, so that he often can hardly stand to be near her. He says he's heard some mention that there is schizophrenia in the family, and wonders if this might be the problem. What could you tell him?

This will require a discussion of the general symptoms and signs of schizophrenia, with specific focus on paranoid schizophrenia.

109. As you enter the cafeteria, you hear two of your friends arguing about the causes of schizophrenia. One is a biology major, who says that the cause is definitely genetic; the other majors in sociology and believes that societal and life-stress factors are the underlying cause. What could you tell your friends about each of their positions, including the types of research that have been done to investigate each? Which position seems more plausible to you?

For the biological basis, this will require a discussion of both the genetic etiology of schizophrenia, together with the different studies that have been done (family studies, twin studies, adoption studies, studies of genetic markers) and the nongenetic biological risks (viral infection, brain structure and function, brain chemistry). The social elements will include a discussion of the psychological risk factors (life-stress, demographic and socioeconomic status, communication and expressed emotion).

110. As you are sitting in the library studying for your next exam in abnormal psychology, you are suddenly startled by a loud disagreement between two students you know. They are arguing about a friend of theirs (someone in one of your classes) who has been institutionalized by his parents. One student says it was the best thing that could have happened, to protect the student from himself. The other says it is totally inhumane, that psychological disorders are merely a means to keep unique people from expressing themselves and that clearly there are other less extreme methods of helping their classmate deal with his problems. Seeing you reading your abnormal psychology text, they ask what you think, especially about committing someone against his or her will, and what is the best way to treat someone who exhibits bizarre behavior. What could you tell them?

This will entail a discussion of treatment, including civil commitment, hospitalization, somatic treatments, and psychological treatments.

111. You have been asked to address a group of mental health volunteers about the symptoms and signs of schizophrenia. They have never before been around people with mental illnesses, and they need some introduction about what they can expect. What could you tell them?

This discussion will include both positive and negative symptoms, with a differentiation between them; it should specifically address, also, the different types of delusions, hallucinations, disorganized speech, behaviors, and affect as well as the aspects of social withdrawal.

112. Imagine that you have not visited your high school since you graduated a few years ago. You return for a class reunion and hear that one of your classmates has been in and out of a mental hospital because she is schizophrenic. Knowing you are majoring in psychology, your former classmates (who have remained in the area and have been friends with this woman) ask you for information about schizophrenia. They want to know how prevalent it is in the population, when people typically get it, what the course of schizophrenia is, and whether your classmate will ever be cured. What could you tell them?

This necessitates a discussion of incidence, prevalence, age of onset (including gender differences); the course of schizophrenia (prodromal phase, active phase, residual phase, the effects of culture); and a discussion of factors that predict outcome.

CHAPTER 10
PERSONALITY AND IMPULSE-CONTROL DISORDERS

MULTIPLE-CHOICE QUESTIONS

1. Experts disagree on all of the following issues concerning personality disorders EXCEPT
   *a. that the behavior is maladaptive and causes anguish.
   b. whether career criminals suffer from a personality disorder or have simply made choices about how to lead their lives.
   c. which personality traits are debilitating enough to be considered a disorder.
   d. that they have very little in common.

   Page: 416   Topic: Introduction

2. All of the following are categorized as impulse-control disorders EXCEPT
   a. fire setting.
   *b. shyness.
   c. gambling.
   d. pulling one's own hair.

   Page: 416   Topic: Introduction

3. The most thoroughly researched personality disorder is
   a. avoidant.
   b. dependent.
   *c. antisocial.
   d. borderline.

   Page: 417   Topic: Introduction

4. In the case of Eric Cooper, the judge who sentenced him believed that
   a. Cooper's criminal behavior was the result of early childhood abuse.
   b. Cooper's criminal behavior was the result of his difficult circumstances.
   c. Cooper had made amends and his victims had forgiven him, so the sentence should be light.
   *d. if people had been less willing to forgive Cooper, his life might have gone differently.

   Page: 418   Topic: Document 10.1: Newspaper Clipping Describing Eric Cooper's Day in Court

5. A person is said to have a personality disorder when
   *a. personality traits produce harmful effects on the person's life.
   b. he or she has problems distinguishing right from wrong.
   c. other people are harmed by the person's behavior.
   d. he or she can no longer distinguish reality.

   Page: 418   Topic: Diagnosing Personality and Impulse-Control Disorders

6. Paul was unable to resist his impulse to set fire to other people's property. He suffers from
   a. kleptomania.
   *b. pyromania.
   c. trichotillomania
   d. arsonomania.

   Page: 418   Topic: Diagnosing Personality and Impulse-Control Disorders

7. All of the following are characteristic of personality disorders EXCEPT:
   a. they begin to become apparent in late childhood or early adolescence.
   b. once they appear, they change little over the years.
   *c. although their roots are in childhood or adolescence, they do not make their first appearance until adulthood.
   d. they affect behavior in numerous situations.

   Page: 418   Topic: Diagnosing Personality and Impulse-Control Disorders

8. Dr. Payne does not like the way the *DSM-IV* categorizes personality disorders because she believes that personality disorders are merely personality traits taken to extremes. Thus, Dr. Payne
   a. believes a person either meets the diagnostic criteria for a personality disorder or does not meet them.
   b. thinks the boundaries between what is normal and what is abnormal are pretty clearly defined.
   c. believes there is no such thing as a personality disorder.
   *d. advocates a dimensional approach.

   Page: 418   Topic: Categories Versus Dimensions

9. Personality disorders are coded on which axis of the *DSM-IV?*
   a. Axis I
   *b. Axis II
   c. Axis III
   d. Axis IV

   Page: 420   Topic: Implications of the Multiaxial Diagnostic System

10. Coding personality disorders on Axis II
    *a. provides a more complex description of a person's problems than would be possible in a single-axis system.
    b. complicates the diagnostic procedure.
    c. simplifies the diagnostic procedure.
    d. is a requirement of insurance companies and health maintenance organizations.

    Page: 420   Topic: Implications of the Multiaxial Diagnostic System

11. As noted in the text, there is a strong link between mood disorders, social phobia, and avoidant personality disorder for all of the following possible reasons EXCEPT:
    a. people with avoidant personalities and social phobias spend too much time alone, which could make them prone to depression.
    b. depression, social phobia, and avoidant personality disorder may share a common etiology.
    *c. people with mood disorders have characteristics that would predispose them to develop social phobias and avoidant personalities.
    d. depression, social phobia, and avoidant personality disorder may be the same condition with different names.

    Page: 422   Topic: Implications of the Multiaxial Diagnostic System

12. Using both Axis I and Axis II provides all of the following diagnostic benefits EXCEPT:
    a. the use of a separate axis for personality disorders reminds clinicians to consider how long-term characterological traits affect the acute symptoms of an Axis I disorder.
    b. Axis II information may be useful in choosing treatment programs.
    c. Axis II information may help in formulating a prognosis for an Axis I disorder.
    *d. the use of a separate axis for clinical disorders simplifies diagnosis if there is no personality disorder present.

    Page: 422   Topic: Implications of the Multiaxial Diagnostic System

13. Inclusion of the 10 personality disorders in the *DSM-IV* is due to
    *a. history and custom.
    b. scientific research.
    c. clinical application.
    d. their greater prevalence than other potential personality disorders.

    Page: 423   Topic: Types of Personality Disorders

14. Linda has been diagnosed with an Axis II personality disorder based on the fact that she exhibits grandiose feelings of superiority. The personality disorder would be
    a. borderline.
    *b. narcissistic.
    c. antisocial.
    d. histrionic.

    Page: 423   Topic: Table 10.2: *DSM-IV* Personality Disorders

15. What sets the impulse-control disorders apart from mere impulsiveness is
    a. the inability to differentiate between right and wrong.
    b. a genetic predisposition.
    *c. a buildup of tension that can be relieved only by acting out the impulse.
    d. a lack of concern for the feelings and rights of others.

    Page: 423   Topic: Types of Impulse-Control Disorders

16. Lupe has bald patches on her scalp, and hair is missing on other parts of her body as well, because she is constantly pulling out her hair. Lupe is suffering from
    a. kleptomania.
    b. pyromania.
    c. hirsutomania.
    *d. trichotillomania.

    Page: 424   Topic: Table 10.3: *DSM-IV* Impulse-Control Disorders

17. A basic problem with diagnosing personality disorders is that
    *a. the same diagnostic criteria apply to different personality disorders.
    b. there is low interrater reliability for the diagnostic criteria.
    c. the diagnostic criteria for the disorders are not clearly defined.
    d. there is little clinical support for most of the diagnostic categories.

    Page: 423   Topic: Diagnostic Reliability

18. When a clinician has to decide whether an impulse-control disorder diagnosis or a personality disorder diagnosis is more appropriate, the *DSM-IV* requires that
    a. the impulse-control diagnosis take precedence.
    *b. the personality disorder diagnosis take precedence.
    c. both diagnoses should be included.
    d. the more clearly distinguished diagnosis take precedence.

    Page: 424   Topic: Diagnostic Reliability

19. Bernie, a pathological gambler, has lost his wife, his children, and his house. After filing for bankruptcy, he was able to get a job that he has kept for the past 4 months. Considering Bernie's personality disorder, what is the best predictor of whether he will gamble?
    a. his past behavior patterns
    b. his health and stress factors
    *c. the social situation in which his behavior takes place
    d. how much child support he owes his wife

    Page: 425   Topic: Diagnostic Validity

20. *Moral insanity,* the precursor to what is now termed *antisocial personality disorder,* attributed criminal behavior to
    a. social conditions.
    b. political conditions.
    c. early childhood training.
    *d. genetics.

    Page: 426   Topic: Evolution of a Personality Disorder: From Psychopath to Antisocial Personality

21. The scientific field that developed in the 19th century to study the causes, prevention, and treatment of criminal behavior is called
    *a. criminology.
    b. criminal psychology.
    c. forensic psychology.
    d. criminal behaviorism.

    Page: 426   Topic: Evolution of a Personality Disorder: From Psychopath to Antisocial Personality

22. The Italian doctor Cesare Lombroso believed that people with inherited moral insanity could be recognized by their
    a. clothing.
    *b. physical features.
    c. behavior.
    d. posture.

    Page: 426   Topic: Psychopaths and Sociopaths

23. The movement away from a genetic explanation for antisocial behavior toward a social explanation
    a. came out of Kraepelin's catetgorizations of behavior.
    b. resulted from the Darwinian influence of evolution.
    *c. was a backlash to the horrors of the Nazi extermination program.
    d. derived from controlled scientific studies of criminal behavior.

    Page: 426   Topic: Psychopaths and Sociopaths

24. The term *psychopath* was changed to *sociopathic personality*
    a. because the latter term better exemplified the characteristics of antisocial behavior.
    b. with the publication of *DSM-II.*
    c. to emphasize antisocial behavior as a personality disorder.
    *d. to signify the dominance of social theories of antisocial behavior.

    Page: 426   Topic: Psychopaths and Sociopaths

25. Eric Cooper, the case study in the text, demonstrated one of the hallmarks of the psychopath. This is
    *a. a flagrant disregard for the rights of others.
    b. the inability to differentiate between right and wrong.
    c. careful planning of actions that are intended to harm others.
    d. a morbid fear of punishment.

    Page: 428   Topic: Psychopaths and Sociopaths

26. In posing the question "Was the president a psychopath?" the text compares Bill Clinton with the psychopaths described by Hervey Cleckley on all of the following characteristics EXCEPT
    a. being charming, intelligent, and engaging.
    *b. demonstrating totally self-centered behavior in his refusal to display contrition.
    c. being unable to resist engaging in high-risk, and ultimately self-defeating, behavior.
    d. initially denying his misbehavior and, when confronted with clear evidence, grudgingly admitting minor wrongdoing.

    Page: 429   Topic: Highlight 10.1: Was the President a Psychopath?

27. For Cleckley, a central clue to the cause of psychopathic behavior is
    a. evidence of early childhood abuse.
    b. finding that other family members are also psychopaths.
    *c. the failure to learn from experience.
    d. a lack of intelligence.

    Page: 429   Topic: Cleckley's Etiological Hypothesis

28. In David Lykken's (1957) experiment comparing psychopaths and nonpsychopaths, he found that
    a. shock was not an effective teaching device for either group.
    b. shock was an effective teaching device for both groups.
    c. shock made no difference to the learning of the nonpsychopathic subjects.
    *d. shock made no difference to the learning of the psychopathic subjects.

    Page: 429   Topic: Cleckley's Etiological Hypothesis

29. In changing the diagnostic categories of *psychopath* and *sociopath* to *antisocial personality disorder,* the *DSM-IV* omitted the concept of
    *a. an inability to feel emotions.
    b. an inability to learn from experience.
    c. a flagrant disregard for the rights and feelings of others.
    d. degree of deviance.

    Page: 430   Topic: *DSM-IV* Abandons Psychopathy

30. The focus of antisocial personality disorder in *DSM-IV,* compared with the previous category of psychopathic behavior, is on
    a. etiological factors.
    *b. observable behaviors.
    c. consequences of behaviors.
    d. observable deviance.

    Page: 430   Topic: *DSM-IV* Abandons Psychopathy

31. The hallmark of the *DSM-IV's* antisocial personality disorder is
    a. an inability to feel emotions.
    b. an inability to learn from experience.
    *c. a flagrant disregard for the rights and feelings of others.
    d. degree of deviance.

    Page: 430   Topic: *DSM-IV* Abandons Psychopathy

32. The *DSM-IV* diagnosis of antisocial personality disorder requires a long-term pattern of all of the following EXCEPT
    a. impulsivity.
    b. aggression.
    c. deception.
    *d. criminality.

    Page: 431   Topic: *DSM-IV* Abandons Psychopathy

33. A *DSM-IV* diagnosis of antisocial personality disorder requires evidence of
    *a. a conduct disorder in childhood.
    b. oppositional defiant disorder in childhood.
    c. a long-term pattern of criminal behavior.
    d. an inability to plan for the future.

    Page: 431   Topic: *DSM-IV* Abandons Psychopathy

34. In the case of Lorena Bobbitt, who cut off her husband's penis while he slept, the court determined that Ms. Bobbitt was
    a. guilty of malicious wounding.
    *b. not guilty by reason of temporary insanity.
    c. not guilty because she was acting in self-defense.
    d. guilty of attempted murder.

    Page: 432   Topic: Critical Thinking About . . . 10.1: Criminal Responsibility: Bad or Mad?

35. The rationale behind an insanity defense requires that people who engage in criminal behavior be divided into two categories. These are
    a. sane and insane.
    b. normal and abnormal.
    *c. bad and mad.
    d. innately bad and innately good.

    Page: 432   Topic: Critical Thinking About . . . 10.1: Criminal Responsibility: Bad or Mad?

36. People who are not responsible for their actions at the time of a crime
    a. are generally acquitted of the crime.
    b. are typically tried for the crime if they understand the nature of the charges against them.
    c. will usually stand trial once they recover sufficiently to participate in their own defense.
    *d. are generally committed for treatment.

    Page: 432   Topic: Critical Thinking About . . . 10.1: Criminal Responsibility: Bad or Mad?

37. The Durham Rule, used by the United States Supreme Court in the 1950s, states that
    *a. any person whose act was the product of a mental disease or mental defect is not criminally responsible for his or her actions.
    b. a person who is unable to resist an impulse, as in a fit of passion, is considered temporarily insane and therefore not guilty of criminal behavior.
    c. a person is insane and not responsible for criminal behavior if the person suffers from a mental disorder and is unable to tell right from wrong.
    d. any person who commits a criminal act, whether sane or insane, will be tried for that criminal act.

    Page: 433   Topic: Critical Thinking About . . . 10.1: Criminal Responsibility: Bad or Mad?

38. With regard to prevalence, who is most likely to be diagnosed with antisocial personality disorder?
    a.   women between the ages of 25 and 44
    *b. men between the ages of 25 and 44
    c.   women over age 44
    d.   men over age 44

    Page: 433   Topic: Prevalence and Course of Antisocial Personality Disorder

39. It is believed that there is a decline in the incidence of antisocial personality disorder in middle and old age for all of the following reasons EXCEPT:
    a.   antisocial personality disorder diminishes with age.
    b.   people with antisocial personality disorder die young from suicide and substance abuse.
    *c. due to age biases, mental health professionals are less likely to diagnose an older person with antisocial personality disorder.
    d.   people with antisocial personality disorder die young from homicide and accidents.

    Page: 433   Topic: Prevalence and Course of Antisocial Personality Disorder

40. In looking for causes of antisocial behavior,
    a.   researchers have found that adopted children grow up to resemble their adoptive parents.
    b.   pedigree studies have identified families with high rates of violent behavior among the female members.
    c.   twin studies have found higher concordance for antisocial traits among fraternal siblings than among nonfraternal siblings.
    *d. twin studies have found higher concordance for antisocial traits among identical siblings than among nonidentical siblings.

    Page: 434   Topic: Genetics

41. The primary reason for withdrawing federal funds for research exploring the link between violence and genetics was
    *a. the belief that genetic research is racially motivated.
    b.   a lack of public interest.
    c.   partisan politics that fought over the best use of the funds.
    d.   the lack of available federal funds to pursue this research.

    Page: 434   Topic: Genetics

42. Research addressing the connection between exposure to violence in the media and aggressive behavior
    a.   has not found a link between the two.
    *b. has found correlations that are too small to explain or predict the violence as a result of media alone.
    c.   has found a strong correlation between exposure to violence in the media and aggressive behavior.
    d.   has found sufficiently strong evidence to assume that exposure to media violence is a causal factor in aggressive behavior.

    Page: 436   Topic: Modeling and Media

43. Dr. Nosital has been studying the etiology of antisocial personality disorder for many years. He agrees with most other experts in the field that the best way to conceptualize our current knowledge of the causes of this disorder is in terms of
    a.   genetic factors.
    b.   sociocultural factors.
    *c. risk factors.
    d.   the media.

    Page: 437   Topic: Causes of Antisocial Personality Disorder: Summary

44. The MOST common treatment for people with antisocial personality disorder is
    a. biological.
    b. psychodynamic.
    c. cognitive-behavioral.
    *d. incarceration.

    Page: 437   Topic: Treatment of Antisocial Personality Disorder

45. Prevention of antisocial personality disorder is typically aimed at
    *a. children and adolescents from high-risk backgrounds.
    b. multimedia exposure in the community.
    c. provision of community resources for young children.
    d. mentoring programs for all school-aged children.

    Page: 437   Topic: Treatment of Antisocial Personality Disorder

46. Potter and Mercy (1997) have found which nation to be the most violent in the industrialized world?
    a. Russia
    *b. the United States
    c. China
    d. Japan

    Page: 440   Topic: Critical Thinking About . . . 10.2: Turbulent Weather Ahead

47. With respect to predicting the probability that a person will commit a violent act, Monahan and Steadman (1996) suggest that psychologists emulate
    a. actuaries.
    b. statisticians.
    *c. meteorologists.
    d. psychics.

    Page: 441   Topic: Critical Thinking About . . . 10.2: Turbulent Weather Ahead

48. If Mario has been diagnosed with one of the Cluster A personality disorders, it would have to be
    a. antisocial or narcissistic.
    b. borderline or histrionic.
    c. avoidant, dependent, or obsessive-compulsive.
    *d. paranoid, schizoid, or schizotypal.

    Page: 439   Topic: Diagnosis, Etiology, and Treatment of the *DSM-IV* Personality Disorders

49. Cluster A personality disorders are marked by
    *a. eccentricity.
    b. self-absorption.
    c. fearfulness.
    d. a tendency toward depression.

    Page: 439   Topic: Cluster A: Paranoid, Schizoid, and Schizotypal Personality Disorders

50. Ted, a brilliant scientist, lives by himself in the woods of Wyoming. He rarely comes into town, and when he does, he appears to be self-absorbed, indifferent, and aloof, clearly not concerned with the opinions of others. Although he appears not to be a happy person, it is somewhat difficult to know for sure because he shows little emotion. Ted likely has which personality disorder?
    a. narcissistic
    *b. schizoid
    c. paranoid
    d. borderline

    Pages: 443–444   Topic: Schizoid Personality Disorder

51. Which type of therapy has proved most effective for persons with schizoid personality disorder?
   a. psychodynamic
   b. cognitive-behavioral
   c. medication
   *d. For most, psychotherapy has not been particularly successful.

   Page: 445   Topic: Schizoid Personality Disorder

52. How does schizotypal personality disorder differ from the schizoid and paranoid personality disorders?
   a. Only the schizotypal personality disorder includes flat affect.
   b. The behavior of persons with paranoid and schizoid personality disorder is more bizarre.
   *c. Only schizotypal personality disorder is related to schizophrenia.
   d. Schizotypal personality disorder is more amenable to treatment.

   Page: 446   Topic: Schizotypal Personality Disorder

53. Clincians and researchers who work from different paradigms have used the term *borderline* in all of the following ways EXCEPT
   *a. as a term for people on the fringes of society who do not have an Axis I disorder.
   b. to refer to people whose behavior falls at some hypothetical border between "neurotic" and "psychotic" mood disorders.
   c. as a general term for the symptoms caused by mild brain damage.
   d. to describe people whose poor social relations are marked by manipulative suicide attempts.

   Page: 447   Topic: Borderline Personality Disorder

54. Miriam demonstrated a relationship pattern in which she would befriend someone and idealize that individual, but would then come to realize that the individual was not perfect and would decide that the person was an enemy. This tendency of people with borderline personality disorder to categorize others as entirely good or entirely bad is known in psychoanalytic circles as
   a. dichotomizing.
   *b. splitting.
   c. shifting.
   d. borderlining.

   Page: 448   Topic: Borderline Personality Disorder

55. Dr. Elofsen is a cognitive-behavioral therapist. In her work with borderline personality disorder she is most likely to use
   a. interpretation of transference.
   b. antianxiety medication.
   *c. dialectical behavior therapy.
   d. skills training.

   Page: 450   Topic: Borderline Personality Disorder

56. Eleanor dresses in rather eccentric, but seductive, clothing. She craves compliments and is easily upset by criticism. She is melodramatic and demands attention. Her personality disorder would be
   a. borderline.
   b. narcissistic.
   c. dependent.
   *d. histrionic.

   Page: 450   Topic: Histrionic Personality Disorder

57. The best therapeutic approach for people with histrionic personality disorder is to help them
   *a. separate important problems from trivial ones and learn to pay attention to others.
    b. develop self-confidence and empathy.
    c. understand that people are not perfect and that it is okay to be human.
    d. learn social skills and problem solving, and to put them on antianxiety medication.

   Page: 451   Topic: Histrionic Personality Disorder

58. Linda appears to have a grandiose sense of her own self-importance, exaggerating her achievements and expecting to be recognized as superior even though her achievements are, at best, mediocre. She believes that she is special and unique and requires constant adulation from the people around her, including her family, clients, boss, and coworkers. Her sense of entitlement has annoyed many coworkers, as have her lack of empathy and constant pattern of taking advantage of others to achieve her goals. Linda has
    a. borderline personality disorder.
   *b. narcissistic personality disorder.
    c. histrionic personality disorder.
    d. antisocial personality disorder.

   Pages: 451–452   Topic: Narcissistic Personality Disorder

59. Jaime is continually seeking assistance, advice, and approval from people he knows. He is rather timid and submissive and seems to be consumed with trying to find someone who will take care of him. Jaime is suffering from _____ personality disorder.
    a. avoidant
    b. histrionic
   *c. dependent
    d. borderline

   Page: 454   Topic: Dependent Personality Disorder

60. People with dependent personality disorder may find their way into therapy
    a. because of the great discomfort they feel.
    b. when other people around them insist they get help.
    c. after being abandoned in several relationships.
   *d. when they seek help for an associated Axis I anxiety or mood disorder.

   Page: 454   Topic: Dependent Personality Disorder

61. "Medicalizing" a behavior by calling it a disorder is justified only when
   *a. doing so leads to some positive outcome, such as prevention, research, or improved functioning.
    b. the disorder clearly is deviant and causes people great discomfort.
    c. the disorder is clearly definable.
    d. enough people seem to have the characteristics that it is worthwhile to classify the behavior.

   Page: 455   Topic: Personality Disorders Under Study

TRUE-FALSE QUESTIONS

62. Taken to extremes, practically any personality trait can impair social functioning and create problems. (T)

   Page: 418   Topic: Diagnosing Personality and Impulse-Control Disorders

63. Some personality disorders do not normally cause an individual personal distress. (T)

   Page: 418   Topic: Diagnosing Personality and Impulse-Control Disorders

64. It is common for a person to be diagnosed as suffering from a clinical disorder on Axis I and a personality disorder on Axis II. (T)

   Page: 420   Topic: Implications of the Multiaxial Diagnostic System

65. An experienced clinician is able to differentiate between the type of impulsivity observed in the impulse-control disorders and the impulsivity found in other disorders. (F)

    Page: 423   Topic: Types of Impulse-Control Disorders

66. Psychopathic people show fewer biological signs of anxiety in the face of potential punishment than do nonpsychopathic people. (T)

    Page: 429   Topic: Cleckley's Etiological Hypothesis

67. The increased objectivity with which the diagnosis of antisocial personality disorder is defined in *DSM-IV* has had a major impact on modern diagnostic practices. (F)

    Page: 430   Topic: *DSM-IV* Abandons Psychopathy

68. In changing the diagnostic category from psychopathy to antisocial personality disorder, the *DSM-IV* narrowed its diagnostic criteria. (F)

    Page: 430   Topic: *DSM-IV* Abandons Psychopathy

69. An antisocial personality is not the equivalent of criminality. (T)

    Page: 431   Topic: *DSM-IV* Abandons Psychopathy

70. The term *insanity* is a psychiatric term. (F)

    Page: 433   Topic: Critical Thinking About . . . 10.1: Criminal Responsibility: Bad or Mad?

71. Antisocial behavior has been found to result from an extra male chromosome. (F)

    Page: 434   Topic: Genetics

72. Studies using modern imaging techniques to examine the brains of delinquent teenagers and antisocial people have not supported the hypothesis that people with antisocial personality disorder are likely to have brain damage to the left hemisphere. (T)

    Page: 434   Topic: Birth Trauma

73. People with antisocial personality disorder may be seeking the stimulation and excitement that come from dangerous behavior as a means to increase their emotional arousal. (T)

    Page: 435   Topic: Sensation Seeking

74. Research indicates that censorship of media violence would significantly reduce violence. (F)

    Page: 437   Topic: Modeling and Media

75. Despite increasing sophistication in measurement devices, psychologists are still not very good at predicting an individual's risk for violent behavior. (T)

    Pages: 440–441   Topic: Critical Thinking About . . . 10.2: Turbulent Weather Ahead

76. There is so much overlap among the Cluster A personality disorders that it is difficult to differentiate them from one another. (T)

    Page: 440   Topic: Cluster A: Paranoid, Schizoid, and Schizotypal Personality Disorders

77. Paranoid personality disorder is a precursor to paranoid schizophrenia. (F)

    Page: 442   Topic: Paranoid Personality Disorder

78. People with schizoid personality disorder rarely seek treatment because they are too disengaged from others to care and too threatened by close relationships to get involved in therapy. (T)

    Page: 444   Topic: Schizoid Personality Disorder

79. According to the *DSM-IV*, people with borderline personality disorder are insecure because they have a morbid fear of abandonment. (T)

    Pages: 447–448   Topic: Borderline Personality Disorder

80. The most effective medications for treatment of borderline personality disorder are the antianxiety drugs. (F)

    Page: 450   Topic: Borderline Personality Disorder

81. Both depressive and passive-aggressive personality disorders will be included in the next edition of the *DSM*. (F)

    Page: 455   Topic: Personality Disorders Under Study

SHORT-ANSWER QUESTIONS

82. Describe the general diagnostic criteria for the personality disorders.

    An enduring pattern of inner experience and behavior that deviates markedly from the expectations of an individual's culture, which is manifested in two or more of the following: cognition, affectivity, interpersonal functioning, and impulse control; the enduring pattern is inflexible and pervasive across a broad range of personal and social situations; the pattern leads to clinically significant distress or impairment in social, occupational, or other important areas of functioning; it is stable and of long duration and its onset can be traced back at least to adolescence or early childhood; it is not better accounted for as a manifestation or consequence of another disorder; and it is not due to the direct physiological effects of a substance or a general medical condition.

    Page: 418   Topic: Diagnosing Personality and Impulse-Control Disorders

83. What are the three types of explanation for the comorbidity between Axis I and Axis II disorders?

    Personality (Axis II) disorders may cause Axis I disorders; both personality and Axis I disorders have a common cause; personality disorders are versions of Axis I disorders.

    Page: 422   Topic: Implications of the Multiaxial Diagnostic System

84. Describe the characteristics of the psychopath, as demonstrated by Eric Cooper, the case study in the text.

    Initially, psychopaths make a good impression because they can be friendly, intelligent, and show no overt signs of mental disorder. However, they have dismal social relationships, disordered work histories, and are often unreliable; they are impulsive; their projects (legal or illegal) turn out badly because they fail to plan ahead; they are self-centered and blame others for their actions but, when pushed, may admit their misdeeds; they feign regret, though their remorse is not genuine and the behavior is repeated; punishment does not deter them, and they engage in actions for which they are likely to be caught.

    Page: 426   Topic: Psychopaths and Sociopaths

85. Outline Cleckley's etiological hypothesis concerning the cause of psychopathic behavior.

    Cleckley hypothesized that the failure to learn from experience was a central clue to the cause of psychopathic behavior. To explain why psychopaths failed to profit from experience, he hypothesized that they are unable to experience normal emotions. They pretend to feel regret, affection, and fear, but they are like actors who simulate emotions they are not really experiencing. Because they do not feel anxiety about future punishment, psychopaths continue to commit antisocial acts for which they have been punished in the past.

    Page: 429   Topic: Cleckley's Etiological Hypothesis

86. Explain the problems in documenting the initial onset of antisocial behavior.

Objective information about a person's childhood is rarely available, retrospective reports by others are often unreliable, and people suspected of being antisocial cannot be trusted to give an accurate history of their own lives.

Pages: 430–431   Topic: *DSM-IV* Abandons Psychopathy

87. What is the M'Naghten Rule, and how did it come about?

The M'Naghten Rule provides that a person is insane, and not responsible for criminal behavior, if the person is suffering from a mental disorder and also is unable to tell right from wrong. It has its origins in 19th-century England when Daniel M'Naghten, while attempting to assassinate the Prime Minister, murdered the Prime Minister's secretary instead. The jury found M'Naghten "not guilty by reason of insanity." The ensuing public outcry led the Law Lords to establish a strict insanity defense, which came to be known as the M'Naghten Rule.

Page: 433   Topic: Critical Thinking About . . . 10.1: Criminal Responsibility: Bad or Mad?

88. Discuss the concerns that have been raised with respect to regional differences in using the insanity defense.

Why should the question of whether a person is insane depend on where he or she lives? Doubts have been raised by disagreement among experts as to who is/is not legally insane. In terms of equity and fairness, if treatment is to be made available, why limit it to those called legally insane—why not make treatment available to everyone with a mental disorder?

Pages: 432–433   Topic: Critical Thinking About . . . 10.1: Criminal Responsibility: Bad or Mad?

89. What are the three primary findings that support a genetic basis for antisocial behavior?

There is a higher concordance for antisocial traits among identical siblings than among nonidentical siblings. Adopted children grow up to resemble their antisocial biological parents more than their non-antisocial adoptive parents; pedigree studies have identified families with high rates of violent behavior among the male members.

Page: 434   Topic: Genetics

90. Explain the family dynamics theory of antisocial personality disorder. What evidence supports this view, and what evidence does not?

The disorder is due to an absence of trust in other people that results from a lack of love during infancy, leading to emotional detachment. Children grow up unable to empathize with others, and, as a result, they become self-absorbed. The evidence for this view is the frequent finding of dysfunctional backgrounds, especially child abuse, in the histories of people with antisocial personality disorder. However, there are many people who grow up with abuse who do not develop the disorder.

Pages: 435–436   Topic: Family Dynamics

91. What are the primary risk factors that would predispose someone to developing antisocial personality disorder?

a poor upbringing combined with exposure to antisocial models (in real life and in the media) and a possible genetic tendency toward low arousal and compensatory sensation-seeking

Page: 437   Topic: Causes of Antisocial Personality Disorder: Summary

92. What are the predominant characteristics of paranoid personality disorder, and what are the consequences of those characteristics?

People with paranoid personality disorder lack trust in others and constantly fear that their friends may be disloyal or unfaithful. As a consequence, they avoid revealing their thoughts and feelings and often are perceived by others as being hypersensitive.

Pages: 440 and 442   Topic: Paranoid Personality Disorder

93. How does paranoid personality disorder different from paranoid schizophrenia?

   Those with paranoid personality disorder do not have delusions, hallucinations, or other forms of thought disorder; instead, they are characterized mainly by their suspicion of other people.

   Pages: 440 and 442   Topic: Paranoid Personality Disorder

94. Describe the similarities between schizotypal personality disorder and schizophrenia.

   Schizotypal personality disorder is most commonly found in families with schizophrenic relatives, and people with schizotypal personality disorder exhibit similar attentional and eye-tracking deficits to people with schizophrenia; both have been linked to higher than average levels of dopamine and to enlarged brain ventricles. Psychotherapy is of limited value in both, with the most successful treatment approaches being skills training and antipsychotic medications.

   Pages: 445–446   Topic: Schizotypal Personality Disorder

95. Contrast the borderline personality with the antisocial personality.

   Both are impulsive, reckless, unable to form stable relationships, and often hostile. The borderline personality is also associated with a morbid fear of abandonment. Men are more likely to be categorized as antisocial and women as borderline.

   Pages: 445–446   Topic: Borderline Personality Disorder

96. Describe passive-aggressive personality disorder and the reason some believe it should not be included in the *DSM*.

   Passive-aggressive personality disorder is characterized by negativistic attitudes and passive resistance to the demands of school and work. Individuals with this disorder habitually resent, oppose, and resist legitimate demands that they function at the level expected of others. They use procrastination, "forget-fulness," stubbornness, and inefficiency to get workmates to shoulder the extra load they shirk. They feel unappreciated and complain about how others treat them and, as a result, are perceived as sullen, irritable, argumentative, cynical, and contrary. Controversy arises over whether these people are simply lazy and also about the stigmatizing effects of labeling.

   Page: 455   Topic: Personality Disorders Under Study

ESSAY QUESTIONS

97. You join your friends for coffee, and one of them says, "I went out with this girl last night, and I couldn't believe it. She had absolutely *no* personality!" The other friend says, "Well, I went on a blind date last night, and I had a dead fish once that had more personality than he had!" Having studied psychology, you know that they are both misusing the term *personality*. What could you tell your friends about what personality is and how to use descriptors more accurately?

   Discuss the definition of personality and how their statements don't fit that definition.

98. Your former high school counselor runs into you at the mall and is delighted to hear that you are taking this class in abnormal psychology. She tells you she would be interested in hearing some of the things you are learning about diagnosing personality and impulse-control disorders. What could you tell her?

   Discuss the various aspects of diagnosing personality and impulse-control disorders, including categories/dimensions, the multiaxial system, types of disorders, and the issues of reliability, validity, and bias.

99. As you come into the student union, you hear some of your classmates from chemistry talking about a recent string of fires that have been set, apparently by one person. They are having a heated debate about what might or might not be wrong with this arsonist. One says the arsonist must have a personality disorder, a second says he's probably a pyromaniac, and a third says he's just a really bad person. Knowing that you are studying abnormal psychology, they turn to you and ask you what would cause someone to behave like this. What could you tell them about personality disorders and impulse-control disorders, as well as about people who are "just bad"? How would the person who is setting the fires be diagnosed according to *DSM-IV?*

   Discuss the personality and impulse-control disorders, differentiate between them, discuss the "mad-versus-bad" literature, and indicate which diagnosis would be suggested by the DSM.

100. As you are reading the newspaper, you note that, after having been arrested for a series of small crimes, one of your childhood schoolmates has just been charged with the cold-blooded murder of a convenience store clerk. The article says that this individual has been diagnosed with antisocial personality disorder. One of your friends looks at the article and asks, "How does someone get that way?" What could you tell your friend?

   Discuss the different theories concerning the etiology of antisocial personality disorder.

101. After you tell your best friend about the various personality disorders, your friend fires a series of questions at you: "How are these people diagnosed? What causes them to be like this? Can they be cured?" What could you tell your friend about the diagnostic criteria, etiology, and treatment of the different personality disorders?

   Discuss diagnostic criteria, etiology, and treatment for each of the three clusters of personality disorders.

CHAPTER 11
INTELLECTUAL AND COGNITIVE DISORDERS

MULTIPLE-CHOICE QUESTIONS

1. The revolution in attitudes toward mental retardation involves
   *a. community-based and school programs replacing custodial institutions.
   b. medications for those with mental retardation that have fewer side effects.
   c. gaining a new understanding of the causes of mental retardation.
   d. using more positive, less pejorative terms to describe people of lower intellectual abilities.

   Page: 460   Topic: Introduction

2. In contrast to mental retardation, the cognitive disorders occur mainly in
   a. early adulthood.
   *b. older people.
   c. children.
   d. adolescents.

   Page: 460   Topic: Introduction

3. A test that estimates the probability that a fetus has one of several birth defects is called a
   _____ test.
   a. prenatal
   b. diagnostic
   *c. screening
   d. family history

   Page: 461   Topic: Document 11.1: Brochure on Genetic Screening . . .

4. A positive prenatal screening test means that the
   a   woman is pregnant.
   b. fetus is healthy.
   c. fetus has one or more birth defects.
   *d. fetus has a higher than average risk for certain birth defects.

   Page: 461   Topic: Document 11.1: Brochure on Genetic Screening . . .

5. A primary risk factor for a child's being born with Down syndrome is the
   *a. mother's age.
   b. father's age.
   c. parents' ethnicity.
   d. mother's pattern of drug use.

   Page: 461   Topic: Helen Lee: A Child With Mental Retardation

6. The Apgar score measures
   a. a baby's mental age.
   *b. a neonate's risk for complications.
   c. the mother's risk factors during birth.
   d. the mother's dilation during labor.

   Page: 462   Topic: Helen Lee: A Child With Mental Retardation

7. Adam is a child with Down syndrome. Based on the characteristic features of the syndrome, we would expect Adam to have all of the following features EXCEPT
    a. a small head and small ears.
    b. a fold of skin that gives his eyes an Asian look.
    *c. long, slender fingers.
    d. a fissured tongue.

    Page: 463   Topic: Helen Lee: A Child With Mental Retardation

8. Prior to 1950, mental retardation was diagnosed on the basis of
    a. an intelligence test.
    b. a battery of psychological tests.
    c. legal precedents.
    *d. a clinical examination.

    Page: 464   Topic: Definition and Diagnosis

9. Sarah is suspected of having Down syndrome. What would be the primary means of assessment?
    *a. an intelligence test
    b. a battery of psychological tests
    c. legal precedents
    d. a clinical examination

    Page: 464   Topic: Definition and Diagnosis

10. Mental retardation is coded on
    a. Axis I.
    *b. Axis II.
    c. Axis III.
    d. Axis IV.

    Page: 464   Topic: Role of Intelligence Tests

11. The overwhelming majority of people with mental retardation are classified under which subtype?
    a. profound
    b. severe
    *c. mild
    d. moderate

    Page: 465   Topic: *DSM-IV* Levels of Mental Retardation and Scores on Intelligence Tests

12. Jason is 27 years old. With an IQ of 45, he requires limited support, can live in a group home, and has learned some skills that allow him to work in a highly supervised capacity. Jason would fall within which subtype of mental retardation?
    a. profound
    b. severe
    c. mild
    *d. moderate

    Page: 465   Topic: *DSM-IV* Levels of Mental Retardation and Scores on Intelligence Tests

13. Understanding that IQ scores are not sufficient to determine a person's ability to function in the world, what other factor has become a critical element of assessment?
    *a. social adaptation
    b. ability to work
    c. family support
    d. mental stability

    Page: 466   Topic: Role of Social Skills

14. With respect to prevalence rates, how is mental retardation related to age?
    a. Prevalence rates are higher in the early years because those who are mentally retarded do not live as long as those of normal intelligence.
    *b. Prevalence rates increase through the school years and decrease in adulthood due to age-related changes in social and intellectual demands.
    c. Prevalence rates decrease through the school years due to the extra attention special needs children receive from the education system.
    d. Prevalence rates remain the same across the life span.

    Page: 468   Topic: How Many People Are Mentally Retarded?

15. If the cutoff point for mental retardation were increased from an IQ of 70 to an IQ of 75, how would that affect the prevalence rate of retardation?
    a. It would stay about the same because retardation has to do with ability to adapt.
    b. Almost 5% of the population would potentially be mentally retarded.
    *c. Almost 10% of the population would potentially be mentally retarded.
    d. Almost 15% of the population would potentially be mentally retarded.

    Page: 469   Topic: Critical Thinking About . . . 11.1: How Many People Do We Want to Be Mentally Retarded?

16. Angel's mental retardation was caused by a genetic condition that made it difficult for him to metabolize a particular amino acid, causing a toxic accumulation in his body that eventually led to his retardation. The metabolic defect that led to Angel's mental retardation is
    a. Down syndrome.
    b. Tay-Sachs disease.
    c. Prader-Willi syndrome.
    *d. phenylketonuria.

    Page: 470   Topic: Inherited Diseases and Genetic Accidents

17. Which of the following describes a way in which a child's environment interacts with a genotype?
    *a. Parents with poor educations who have a child with PKU must understand the labels on food products.
    b. Poor children living in old or substandard housing are likely to eat paint chips that contain lead.
    c. A mother over age 35 is at high risk for giving birth to a child with Down syndrome.
    d. Jewish parents of Eastern European ancestry are at high risk for having a child with Tay-Sachs disease.

    Page: 470   Topic: Inherited Diseases and Genetic Accidents

18. Which metabolic disorder will show up in a child only if both parents are carriers?
    a. phenylketonuria
    *b. Niemann-Pick
    c. trisomy 21
    d. fragile X syndrome

    Page: 470   Topic: Inherited Diseases and Genetic Accidents

19. Down syndrome is the result of
    a. phenylketonuria.
    b. Niemann-Pick.
    *c. trisomy 21.
    d. fragile X syndrome.

    Page: 470   Topic: Inherited Diseases and Genetic Accidents

20. Because the amount of _____ varies from person to person, a wide range of mental retardation and developmental delay is noted among children with Down syndrome.
    a. genetic material
    b. chromosomes
    c. protein
    *d. overexpression

    Page: 470   Topic: Inherited Diseases and Genetic Accidents

21. A genetic disorder resulting in mild to severe mental retardation caused by part of a chromosome being replicated many times, so that affected individuals may have more than 1,000 copies of a particular genetic string, is
    *a. fragile X syndrome.
    b. Turner's syndrome.
    c. Klinefelter's syndrome.
    d. cri du chat syndrome.

    Page: 471   Topic: Inherited Diseases and Genetic Accidents

22. Ten-year-old Viola has a pixielike, narrow face with a broad forehead, wide-spaced eyes, and a sharp chin. She appears to be a child prodigy when it comes to music and has already won several competitions for her virtuosity in playing the violin. However, she cannot tie her shoes, and often when she speaks, no one can understand her, although her speech is fluent. Viola suffers from
    a. Prader-Willi syndrome.
    *b. Williams syndrome.
    c. Klinefelter's syndrome.
    d. Down syndrome.

    Page: 471   Topic: Inherited Diseases and Genetic Accidents

23. Teratogenic agents affect a child's development at any time during the
    a. entire childhood period.
    b. first year of life.
    c. first month of life.
    *d. mother's pregnancy.

    Page: 472   Topic: Pregnancy Complications, Birth Trauma, and Childhood Problems: Teratogenic Agents

24. Prenatal infections that can cause mental retardation in children could be eliminated by
    a. proper screening.
    b. diagnostic techniques.
    *c. vaccinations and use of condoms.
    d. appropriate diet and exercise.

    Page: 473   Topic: Pregnancy Complications, Birth Trauma, and Childhood Problems: Prenatal Infection

25. What is the relationship between birth weight and IQ?
    a. Low-birth-weight children have higher IQs than normal-birth-weight children.
    b. Low-birth-weight children have lower IQs than normal-birth-weight children.
    *c. Both low-birth-weight and high-birth-weight children have lower IQs than normal-birth-weight children.
    d. There is no relationship between birth weight and IQ.

    Page: 474   Topic: Prematurity

26. Most mild cases of mental retardation are considered to be _____ in origin.
    a. genetic
    b. environmental
    c. sociocultural
    *d. cultural-familial
    Page: 474   Topic: Cultural-Familial Factors

27. Studies of adopted children have found that their IQ scores correlate with the educational levels and IQs of their
    *a. biological mothers.
    b. adoptive mothers.
    c. foster mothers.
    d. biological fathers.
    Page: 475   Topic: Cultural-Familial Factors

28. A cause of ambiguity in twin studies examining the concordance rate for intelligence of twins raised apart from birth is that:
    a. not all identical twins have similar IQs.
    *b. separated twins are often raised by relatives, who provide similar environments.
    c. most of the studies done on twins separated at birth have methodological flaws.
    d. several of the researchers studying identical twins have altered their data.
    Page: 475   Topic: Cultural-Familial Factors

29. The neglect of _____ is a major omission in the research on the heritability of intelligence.
    a. intelligence test scores
    b. personality test scores
    *c. adaptive behavior
    d. academic performance
    Page: 475   Topic: Cultural-Familial Factors

30. Adopted children may have higher IQs than their biological mothers because
    a. adopted children are more likely to resemble their adoptive mothers than their biological mothers.
    b. the statistical methods used to analyze these relationships produce spurious results.
    c. environment has a stronger influence on children's intelligence than heredity.
    *d. adoptive families may provide stimulating intellectual environments that allow the children to reach their intellectual potential.
    Page: 476   Topic: Highlight 11.1: Biology Is Not Quite Destiny

31. The term *learning disabilities* includes all of the following EXCEPT _____ disorders.
    *a. adaptability
    b. learning
    c. communication
    d. motor skills
    Page: 475   Topic: Origins

32. Paul Broca (1861) was a pioneer in the field of learning disabilities due to his
    a. discovery of brain defects responsible for a wide array of cognitive disabilities.
    *b. observation that language disorders are correlated with damage to the left cerebral hemisphere.
    c. discovery of several brain sites involved in language functioning.
    d. observations of school children who were having difficulties learning to read, write, and do arithmetic.
    Page: 476   Topic: Origins

33. When autopsies of dyslexic people revealed no visible brain damage, clinicians
    a. abandoned the theory that dyslexia is the result of brain damage.
    b. amended the theory of the etiology of dyslexia to include environmental factors as well.
    *c. assumed that the damage was not visible on autopsy.
    d. determined that there must be some other cause of dyslexia.

    Pages: 476–477   Topic: Origins

34. Helen Lee, the case study in the text, was not diagnosed with a learning disorder because
    a. the diagnosis of mental retardation took precedence over the diagnosis of a learning disorder.
    b. her retardation was so severe as to render her untestable.
    c. she had visual and auditory deficits that ruled out a diagnosis of learning disorder.
    *d. her skills were not substantially below the level expected for her age, schooling, and intelligence.

    Page: 477   Topic: Diagnosis

35. Mary has a history of failure to use speech sounds appropriately, often substituting one sound for another and making many pronunciation errors. She has which type of learning disorder?
    *a. phonological disorder
    b. expressive language disorder
    c. mixed receptive-expressive language disorder
    d. stuttering

    Page: 479   Topic: Table 11.4: *DSM-IV* Diagnostic Criteria for Learning, Motor, and Communication Disorders

36. Who of the following was considered mentally retarded as a child by his parents and his teachers?
    a. Albert Einstein
    *b. Thomas Edison
    c. Sigmund Freud
    d. Benjamin Franklin

    Page: 478   Topic: Highlight 11.2: Smart People May Have Troubles, Too

37. Lewis Terman's longitudinal study of California school children with IQ scores over 135 has found that
    a. a very large number of participants in the research became mentally ill.
    b. the study participants showed poorer adjustment than the average population.
    *c. the study participants showed better adjustment than the average population.
    d. there is no relationship between intelligence and adjustment or mental illness.

    Page: 478   Topic: Highlight 11.2: Smart People May Have Troubles, Too

38. Most learning disabilities affect
    a. children who are mentally retarded.
    b. both boys and girls equally.
    c. girls more often than boys.
    *d. boys more often than girls.

    Page: 477   Topic: Causes

39. What is the relationship between learning disabilities and mental illness?
    *a. There is a high correlation between learning disabilities, depression, and adolescent suicide.
    b. Learning disabilities often lead to depression and adolescent suicide.
    c. The vulnerability that leads to learning disabilities also leads to depression and adolescent suicide.
    d. There is no relationship between learning disabilities and any mental illness.

    Page: 477   Topic: Causes

40. The driving force behind deinstitutionalization and returning people with mental retardation back into the community was
    a. economics.
    *b. normalization.
    c. politics.
    d. humanism.

    Page: 478   Topic: Treating Mental Retardation and Learning Disabilities

41. Today, most mentally retarded children live
    a. in institutions.
    b. in community-based facilities.
    *c. at home.
    d. in boarding schools.

    Page: 479   Topic: Treating Mental Retardation and Learning Disabilities

42. Educational goals for children who are moderately retarded focus mainly on
    a. remedial academic subjects.
    b. overcoming their disorder.
    c. pushing them toward the top of their intellectual range.
    *d. self-help skills.

    Page: 479   Topic: Treating Mental Retardation and Learning Disabilities

43. An educational approach that seems to help children learn, which includes strategies such as teaching in novel ways, is called
    *a. scaffolding.
    b. the jigsaw approach.
    c. mainstreaming.
    d. strategizing.

    Page: 480   Topic: Treating Mental Retardation and Learning Disabilities

44. With respect to mainstreaming, the text suggests that the best option for most students who are mentally retarded or learning disabled is to
    a. home-school them.
    *b provide segregated instruction when necessary and integrate them into normal classrooms when possible.
    c. mainstream them into the normal classroom.
    d. provide special classes where they receive individual attention.

    Page: 481   Topic: Treating Mental Retardation and Learning Disabilities

45. The story about Richard Lapointe, who, on the basis of his signed confession, was convicted of raping and murdering his wife's grandmother, underscores all of the following EXCEPT the
    a. abuses of police interrogations.
    b. importance of taped interrogations.
    *c. criminal tendencies of people who are mentally retarded.
    d. need to teach lawyers and judges about mental retardation.

    Page: 483   Topic: Highlight 11.3: Justice for All?

46. Based on an examination of the case histories of 2,000 full-time residents of institutions for people with mental retardation, Stevenson and his colleagues (1996) estimated that, if all primary prevention strategies were used, the prevalence of severe and profound mental retardation could be reduced by
_____%.
   a. 5
   b. 10
   c. 15
*d. 20

   Page: 481   Topic: Primary and Secondary Prevention

47. All of the following are primary prevention strategies aimed at reducing the prevalence of severe and profound mental retardation EXCEPT
*a. exposure to stimulation programs.
   b. genetic screening and counseling.
   c. immunization.
   d. elimination of potential teratogenic agents.

   Page: 481   Topic: Primary and Secondary Prevention

48. Tertiary prevention programs for those with mental retardation are aimed at
   a. prolonging their lives and keeping them healthy.
*b. preventing deterioration and maintaining as high a functional level as possible for independent living.
   c. providing financial and emotional support.
   d. dealing with their ongoing social, medical, and educational needs.

   Page: 482   Topic: Tertiary Prevention

49. Twenty-year-old Sheldon has benefited from the current wave of supported employment initiatives. As a result,
   a. his parents are able to alternate taking him to work with them.
   b. day care facilities are available at his parents' places of employment where Sheldon can be cared for while his parents work.
*c. adjustments have been made to the workplace so that Sheldon can now engage in productive employment.
   d. more menial jobs have opened up for those who are mentally retarded, which means that Sheldon can be paid to do simple tasks.

   Pages: 482–483   Topic: Tertiary Prevention

50. A particularly common degenerative brain disorder among people with Down syndrome is
   a. vascular dementia.
   b. Parkinson's disease.
   c. Creutzfeldt-Jakob disease.
*d. dementia of the Alzheimer's type.

   Page: 484   Topic: Helen Lee: An Adult With Mental Retardation

51. Rogelio hears doors banging open and shut and sees skeleton heads pop out of windows, although no one around him experiences these events. He is typically disoriented, often forgets his own name, and seems to be in a fog. From which cognitive disorder is Rogelio suffering?
*a delirium
   b. dementia
   c. Alzheimer's
   d. amnestic disorders

   Page: 485   Topic: Main *DSM-IV* Cognitive Disorders

52. What did Esquirol believe to be the cause of what he termed *chronic dementia?*
    a. fever or hemorrhage
    *b. drunkenness or masturbation
    c. disease or a blow to the head
    d. old age

    Page: 485   Topic: Dementia and the Other Cognitive Disorders

53. Mgumbe's doctor suspected he had a brain tumor, and thus ordered a series of tests. One test, the
    _____, involved the administration of a radioactive form of glucose that resulted in an image of
    the metabolic activity in different parts of Mgumbe's brain as Mgumbe performed a variety of cognitive
    tasks.
    a. computerized tomography (CT) scan
    b. magnetic resonance imaging (MRI)
    *c. positron emission tomography (PET) scan
    d. single photon emission computerized tomography (SPECT) scan

    Pages: 488–489   Topic: Highlight 11.4: Seeing Inside the Brain

54. In addition to memory impairment, the *DSM-IV* requires any of the following EXCEPT _____
    for a diagnosis of dementia.
    a. agnosia
    b. aphasia
    c. apraxia
    *d. echolalia

    Page: 486   Topic: Diagnosing Dementia

55. Eduardo has been having trouble recognizing common items that he has known all his life, such as apples,
    keys, and forks. Eduardo is exhibiting
    *a. agnosia.
    b. aphasia.
    c. apraxia.
    d. echolalia.

    Page: 486   Topic: Diagnosing Dementia

56. Delirium, a cognitive disorder marked by a clouding of consciousness,
    a. is most commonly seen in young adults.
    *b. develops rapidly.
    c. is present in close to 25% of emergency room patients.
    d. rarely occurs in people who have not been heavy drinkers.

    Page: 487   Topic: Ruling Out Delirium and Depression

57. Depression can be differentiated from dementia in all of the following ways EXCEPT:
    a. depressive episodes have at least a vague beginning and an end, whereas dementia develops too
       gradually to pinpoint a date.
    b. depressed people are aware of and complain about their cognitive functioning and most respond to
       antidepressant medication.
    *c. depressed people withdraw from their normal activities and lose interest in everyday life, whereas
       people with dementia only do this in the late stages of the disorder.
    d. the symptoms of depression are usually worse in the morning, whereas dementia symptoms become
       more obvious late in the day.

    Pages: 489–490   Topic: Ruling Out Delirium and Depression

58. David has been diagnosed with dementia as the result of a stroke. This is called:
    a. dementia of the Alzheimer's type.
    b. substance-induced persisting dementia.
    c. dementia due to medical conditions.
    *d. vascular dementia.

    Page: 490   Topic: Vascular Dementia

59. Parkinson's disease is associated with a type of dementia characterized by symptoms of psychomotor slowness and a memory deficit called
    *a. subcortical dementia.
    b. vascular dementia.
    c. neural dementia.
    d. Pick's disease.

    Page: 491   Topic: Parkinson's Disease

60. Arnold's dementia is caused by the atrophy of the frontal and temporal lobes of his brain. In addition to cognitive impairments, he also displays behaviors characteristic of frontal lobe damage, especially disinhibition. Arnold has
    a. Parkinson's disease.
    *b. Pick's disease.
    c. Huntington's disease.
    d. Creutzfeldt-Jakob disease.

    Page: 492   Topic: Pick's Disease

61. Woody Guthrie, one of America's most prolific folk musicians, first experienced mild memory impairment, an inability to concentrate, and depression; then personality changes. As his disease progressed, his cognitive impairments became more noticeable, and his movements became jerky and irregular. He was afflicted with
    a. Parkinson's disease.
    b. Pick's disease.
    *c. Huntington's disease.
    d. Creutzfeldt-Jakob disease.

    Page: 492   Topic: Huntington's Disease

62. Many members of the Fore tribe of Papua New Guinea have developed a slow-growing virus called kuru that is
    a. genetically transmitted.
    b. the result of eating infected cattle.
    c. transmitted by local insects.
    *d. transmitted by eating the dead bodies of other tribe members.

    Page: 493   Topic: Creutzfeldt-Jakob Disease

63. Phineas sustained damage to his frontal lobe. We would expect to see all of the following behavioral effects EXCEPT
    *a. an inability to recognize familiar objects.
    b. disinhibition.
    c. memory deficit.
    d. a loss of abstract reasoning.

    Pages: 493–494   Topic: Head Injuries, Tumors, and Other Brain Diseases

64. After the death of a 55-year-old patient whom he had diagnosed with senile dementia, Alois Alzheimer found all of the following EXCEPT
    a. neurofibrillary tangles.
    *b. atherosclerosis.
    c. senile plaques.
    d. arteriosclerosis.

    Page: 494   Topic: Dementia of the Alzheimer's Type

65. Today Alzheimer's is diagnosed when
    a. neurofibrillary tangles and senile plaques are found on autopsy.
    b. an MRI or a CT scan exhibits atrophy in major areas of the brain.
    *c. all other types of dementia have been ruled out.
    d. the behaviors and brain scans fit the profile researchers have developed.

    Page: 495   Topic: Dementia of the Alzheimer's Type

66. The prevalence rate of Alzheimer's for people in their late 80s is
    a. 1%.
    b. 5%.
    c. 8%.
    *d. 10%.

    Page: 495   Topic: Prevalence, Incidence, and Course of Dementia

67. What is the relationship between cigarette smoking and Alzheimer's?
    *a. Although smokers seem to have lower rates of Alzheimer's, it may be because they die before it has a chance to develop.
    b. People who smoke cigarettes have a greater chance of developing Alzheimer's than people who don't because smoking reduces oxygen to the brain.
    c. People who smoke cigarettes have a reduced risk of developing Alzheimer's due to the protective factors of nicotine.
    d. There is no relationship between cigarette smoking and developing Alzheimer's.

    Page: 496   Topic: Risk Factors for and Etiology of Dementia

68. What have researchers determined concerning the heritability of Alzheimer's?
    a. Twin studies have found higher concordance rates for Alzheimer's among dizygotic twins than among monozygotic twins.
    *b. The genetic data may be interpreted to suggest that it is not Alzheimer's that is inherited, but the tendency to live long enough to be symptomatic.
    c. Familial Alzheimer's is characterized by a later age of onset and slower deterioration.
    d. Adoption studies have demonstrated that a person is more likely to develop Alzheimer's if his or her biological parents had the disease.

    Pages: 496–497   Topic: Risk Factors for and Etiology of Dementia

69. Eve has an amnestic disorder. We would expect her to be able to do all of the following EXCEPT
    a. pay attention to her immediate situation.
    b. retrieve old memories.
    *c. learn new information.
    d. repeat a list of four or five digits.

    Page: 497   Topic: Amnestic Disorders

70. Sergei was diagnosed with Korsakoff's syndrome. His disorder was caused by
    a. a genetic disorder that predisposed him to a vitamin B_{12} deficiency because of his inability to metabolize food.
    b. severe head trauma and chronic substance abuse.
    c. an anomaly in the 13th pair of chromosomes that affects his testosterone levels.
    *d. the poisoning of nerve cells by alcohol and a vitamin B_1 deficiency caused by poor diet.

    Page: 498   Topic: Amnestic Disorders

71. The most common treatment for Alzheimer's today is
    *a. donepezil hydrochloride (Aricept).
    b. tacrine hydrochloride (Cognex).
    c. Thyroxin.
    d. L-dopa.

    Page: 498   Topic: Amnestic Disorders

72. The aims of treatment for dementia include all of the following EXCEPT
    a. preserving the person's sense of independence and self-esteem.
    *b. prolonging the person's life.
    c. helping the person keep up social contacts.
    d. providing the person with as much enjoyment and meaning in life as possible.

    Pages: 498–499   Topic: Amnestic Disorders

73. People who are considered legally incompetent
    a. are nonetheless liable for their criminal behavior.
    b. retain the right to refuse medical treatment.
    *c. lose their personal autonomy.
    d. may chose to change their legal guardian in the event of an irreconcilable dispute.

    Page: 500   Topic: Legal Implications of Intellectual and Cognitive Disorders

74. Anne wishes to avoid the need for her children to make life-choice decisions for her in the event she is no longer capable of making those decisions herself. Her best option would be to _____ while she is still legally competent.
    a. tell her grandchildren what should be done on her behalf
    b. put detailed instructions in her will
    c. prepare a living trust to see to her needs
    *d. prepare a living will stating when to discontinue medical treatment

    Page: 500   Topic: Legal Implications of Intellectual and Cognitive Disorders

TRUE-FALSE QUESTIONS

75. If a prenatal screening test is negative, it means that the baby will not have a birth defect. (F)

    Page: 461   Topic: Document 11.1: Brochure on Genetic Screening . . .

76. The number of people in the profound range of mental retardation exceeds what we would expect on a purely statistical basis. (T)

    Page: 464   Topic: Role of Intelligence Tests

77. Low intelligence (below an IQ of 70) is sufficient for a diagnosis of mental retardation. (F)

    Page: 466   Topic: Role of Social Skills

78. Interventions aimed at improving adaptive skills can reduce the prevalence of mental retardation. (T)

    Page: 468   Topic: Critical Thinking About . . . 11.1: How Many People Do We Want to Be Mentally Retarded?

79. The most definitive studies concerning the heritability of intelligence come from the research of Sir Cyril Burt. (F)

    Page: 475   Topic: Cultural-Familial Factors

80. Adaptive behavior is inherited in the same way as intelligence is. (F)

    Page: 475   Topic: Cultural-Familial Factors

81. If a person who is mentally retarded scores low for his or her age on learning, motor skills, and language abilities, but not lower than what might be expected considering his or her level of retardation, then that person will not be diagnosed with a learning disability. (T)

    Page: 477   Topic: Diagnosis

82. Most gifted people were precocious children. (F)

    Page: 478   Topic: Highlight 11.2: Smart People May Have Troubles, Too

83. Teaching students who are mentally retarded or who have learning disabilities to use sign language can help them learn other forms of communication. (T)

    Page: 480   Topic: Treating Mental Retardation and Learning Disabilities

84. The best option for most students who are mentally retarded or learning disabled is to be mainstreamed into normal classes. (F)

    Page: 481   Topic: Treating Mental Retardation and Learning Disabilities

85. Cognitive disorders are always the result of neurological dysfunction. (T)

    Page: 484   Topic: Dementia and the Other Cognitive Disorders

86. Dementia is more common today than it was in previous periods of time. (T)

    Page: 485   Topic: Dementia and the Other Cognitive Disorders

87. Positron emission tomography (PET) scans can provide images of brain structure. (F)

    Page: 488   Topic: Highlight 11.4: Seeing Inside the Brain

88. The safest technique for examining the brain is the positron emission tomography (PET) scan. (F)

    Page: 488   Topic: Highlight 11.4: Seeing Inside the Brain

89. Not knowing one's birthday may be a sign of cognitive impairment. (T)

    Page: 487   Topic: Diagnosing Dementia

90. The symptoms of depression and dementia are sufficiently similar to make a differential diagnosis extremely difficult. (T)

    Page: 489   Topic: Ruling Out Delirium and Depression

91. The huge body of research, first stimulated by Kraepelin, has ultimately substantiated his distinction between presenile and old-age dementia. (F)

    Page: 494   Topic: Dementia of the Alzheimer's Type

92. Neurofibrillary tangles and senile plaques are common in old people who have no symptoms of dementia. (T)

    Page: 495   Topic: Dementia of the Alzheimer's Type

93. Research evidence supports the suggestion that aluminum is a risk factor for developing Alzheimer's. (F)

    Page: 496   Topic: Risk Factors for and Etiology of Dementia

94. The best way to ensure that your wishes concerning discontinuation of medical treatment are carried out in the event you become legally incompetent is to prepare a living will. (T)

    Page: 500   Topic: Legal Implications of Intellectual and Cognitive Disorders

SHORT-ANSWER QUESTIONS

95. What are the three decisions a pregnant woman over age 35 would need to make in terms of prenatal testing?

    whether she wants a screening test; if the screening test is positive, whether to undergo a diagnostic test; if the diagnostic test shows the fetus to have a birth defect, whether to terminate the pregnancy

    Pages: 460–461   Topic: Document 11.1: Brochure on Genetic Screening . . .

96. Describe the problems with using intelligence tests to assess mental retardation.

    Although intelligence tests were introduced to make intellectual assessments more objective, they are not neutral measures. People with certain disabilities (such as hearing impairment) may be inappropriately classified unless special testing arrangements are made to accommodate their physical needs. Also, racial and ethnic biases in the testing instruments produce lower scores for African American and Latino children, so they are overdiagnosed relative to their numbers in the population. Calling members of these groups mentally retarded stigmatizes them and makes retardation at least partly a racial and ethnic phenomenon when, in reality, low scores likely reflect group members' social and economic deprivation.

    Pages: 464–465   Topic: Role of Intelligence Tests

97. Discuss the social and economic issues involved in raising the IQ cutoff point for a determination of mental retardation.

    Classifying more people as mentally retarded might make more people eligible for special education and thus give them a brighter future; however, society would incur the costs of providing special education to more students. If society is willing to spend more money on education, then a higher cutoff may be justified; if we want to economize, then a lower cutoff will save money and also limit the number potentially stigmatized by being labeled retarded.

    Page: 469   Topic: How Many People Do We Want to Be Mentally Retarded?

98. Categorize and give examples of the five main causes of mental retardation.

    The five causes are genetic, including inherited conditions, genetic accidents, and mutations caused by exposure to X rays or other toxins; pregnancy complications, caused by alcohol, drug poisoning, or illness; birth trauma, caused by anoxia or stressful delivery; childhood diseases or accidents; and social factors, such as poverty, poor nutrition, child abuse, or a deprived intellectual environment.

    Page: 469   Topic: Causes

99. What are the eight specific disorders included in the learning disabilities, and what is the *general* diagnostic criterion?

   The disorders are reading disorder, mathematics disorder, disorder of written expression, motor skills disorder, expressive language disorder, mixed receptive-expressive language disorder, phonological disorder, and stuttering. For each of the disorders, the disturbance must significantly interfere with academic or occupational achievement or some area of social life; if mental retardation or a sensory defect is present, then the disturbance must be greater than those usually associated with these conditions.

   Page: 479   Topic: Table 11.4: *DSM-IV* Diagnostic Criteria for Learning, Motor, and Communication Disorders

100. Describe what scaffolding is and some of the techniques that are used.

   Scaffolding provides students with an assistive framework (a "scaffold") from which to learn. Strategies include teaching in novel ways so that students who would not learn well using the normal methods can perform at a higher level: for example, teaching rudimentary sign language to help a child communicate with parents and teachers, as well as "assistive technologies" such as the spell checkers and grammar checkers in computerized word-processing programs, speech synthesizers for students with reading disorders, and talking calculators for students with mathematics disorder.

   Pages: 478–481   Topic: Treating Mental Retardation and Learning Disabilities

101. Identify the primary prevention strategies that could serve to reduce the prevalence of mental retardation.

   genetic screening and counseling; immunization; the elimination of potential teratogenic agents

   Page: 481   Topic: Primary and Secondary Prevention

102. What are the three possible causes of cognitive disorders?

   a general medical condition; a substance (drug or toxin); a combination of both

   Pages: 484–485   Topic: Dementia and the Other Cognitive Disorders

103. Describe the three main cognitive disorders delineated in the *DSM-IV.*

   Dementia: Multiple cognitive deficits including forgetfulness, disorientation, concrete thinking, and perseveration. Delirium: Cloudy consciousness accompanied by disorientation, memory deficits, perceptual disturbances such as hallucinations, and language deficits. Amnestic disorders: Loss of past memories or an inability to learn new information.

   Page: 484   Topic: Dementia and the Other Cognitive Disorders

104. Describe the different brain imaging techniques that scientists use to examine the structure and function of the living brain.

   Computerized tomography (CT) scans use multiple beams of X rays that revolve around the head, transmitting a computer-analyzed cross-sectional image of the brain that shows the outlines of certain brain structures. Magnetic resonance imaging (MRI) uses powerful magnetic fields to attract the protons in the nuclei of the body's hydrogen atoms, changing their alignment to give off radio transmissions that are translated into images of the brain. Positron emission tomography (PET) scans reveal brain function by administering radioactive glucose that is metabolized in active brain cells to identify the parts of the brain that are active during certain cognitive tasks. Electroencephalographic (EEG) methods record the brain's electrical activity; by recording which areas of the brain are responding to specific stimuli, researchers can construct a topographic map representing electrical activity in various parts of the brain. Single photon emission computerized tomography (SPECT) scans produce topographic maps of the brain by monitoring blood flow while people perform cognitive tasks.

   Page: 488   Topic: Highlight 11.4: Seeing Inside the Brain

105. Describe the diagnostic requirements for dementia.

The DSM-IV requires that these include a memory impairment and one or more of the following symptoms: aphasia (a language disorder usually associated with damage to the left cerebral hemisphere), agnosia (a failure to recognize familiar objects despite normal vision, touch, and hearing), and apraxia (an inability to carry out desired motor actions despite normal muscle control).

Pages: 486–487   Topic: Diagnosing Dementia

106. What are the steps in diagnosing dementia?

First, the clinician must confirm that the person suffers from multiple cognitive deficits. Second, the clinician must determine, on the basis of the client's family and medical history, whether the observed cognitive deficits are lifelong or acquired because, by definition, dementia is acquired. Third, the clinician must rule out conditions that are superficially similar to dementia, such as delirium or depression.

Pages: 486–487   Topic: Diagnosing Dementia

107. Describe the course of dementia of the Alzheimer's type.

Both early- and late-onset cases usually begin with a mild memory disturbance that is often dismissed as mere forgetfulness. As time passes, the memory disturbance becomes more obvious. Not only does the person forget facts and events, but new learning becomes increasingly difficult. Initially, old memories are preserved, but eventually those, too, are lost. Personality changes, sometimes dramatic, come next. People with dementia become childish, irritable, and depressed, which is followed by increasing confusion, disorientation, aphasia, agnosia, and apraxia. In the late stages, people may lose control over body functions. Death usually follows soon after.

Page: 495   Topic: Prevalence, Incidence, and Course of Dementia

108. Describe the modifications to home environment and daily routine that help foster a sense of independence and control for someone suffering from dementia or an amnestic disorder.

Hand rails permit a person with apraxia to get around the house and to use the bathroom without assistance; special chairs and beds that make it easy to sit, lie down, and rise, and remote controls that permit the television to be operated from a distance help promote independence; printed labels or pictures on cupboard doors help people with memory disorders to locate common household items; colored arrows drawn on floors help people navigate around their homes without getting lost; strategically placed reminders can help people to function more or less independently. Community services, such as meal preparation and visiting nurses, allow many people who would otherwise need institutional care to live at home.

Pages: 498–499   Topic: Treatment and Prevention of Cognitive Disorders

109. What is a living will, and why would someone want to prepare one?

A living will, which is accepted in most jurisdictions, contains advance directives stipulating when medical treatment should be discontinued. It is prepared when a person is still legally competent, in order to preempt the authority of guardians and ensure that the person's own wishes are followed with respect to medical treatment and continuation/discontinuation of life.

Page: 500   Topic: Legal Implications of Intellectual and Cognitive Disorders

ESSAY QUESTIONS

110. One of your classmates from another class confides in you that he has a learning disability. He tells you that people have called him a "retard" his whole life. He knows you are taking this class in abnormal psychology and asks you to tell him the difference between being "retarded" and having a learning disability. What information could you share with him?

Compare and contrast mental retardation and learning disabilities.

111. Knowing that you are a psychology major and that you are taking this class in abnormal psychology, one of your neighbors asks for your help with two problems. For one thing, she tells you her daughter was born with Down syndrome. Also, her mother died a few years ago, and now her aging father will be moving in with her and her family, and he has Alzheimer's. She asks you for advice on providing the optimum environment for her daughter, her father, and the rest of the family. What could you advise her?

Discuss the various treatments available for mental retardation and the issues involved in maximizing each individual's potential, including issues of mainstreaming; then address the treatments for dementia and ways to design and use the environment to provide the maximum amount of independence.

112. Your favorite elementary school counselor, with whom you have kept in touch all these years, has asked you to sit on a panel to discuss how we can prevent intellectual and cognitive disorders from affecting people in the future. What could you say on this panel?

Discuss primary, secondary, and tertiary prevention for mental retardation and learning disabilities, as well as the known risk factors for dementia, providing suggestions on how to reduce the risk factors for all intellectual and cognitive disorders.

113. Your parents and grandparents are beginning to consider the possibility that their mental and physical health will, at some point, begin to decline. They want to do the very best for the family, so they decide to have a family meeting to discuss the legal implications of intellectual and cognitive disorders. What specific issues should be part of this discussion?

Discuss the legal implications of intellectual and cognitive disorders, being sure to address legal competence and living wills.

114. A homeless man you know was recently arrested by the police and accused of raping a young woman. The police say the man has confessed to the crime, but you know the man is moderately retarded. What issues would be important in determining this man's guilt or innocence?

Discuss the potential abuses of civil rights that may occur during police interrogation and how those abuses may be ended.

CHAPTER 12
DISORDERS OF CHILDHOOD AND ADOLESCENCE

MULTIPLE-CHOICE QUESTIONS

1. As a _____, Dr. Williamson would study abnormal behavior in its developmental context.
   *a. developmental psychopathologist
   b. child developmentalist
   c. developmental psychologist
   d. school counselor

   Page: 506   Topic: Introduction

2. Which of the following disorders are usually first noticed in childhood or adolescence?
   a. unipolar and bipolar disorder
   *b. enuresis and oppositional defiant disorder
   c. antisocial personality disorder and dependent personality disorder
   d. schizophrenia and dissociative identity disorder

   Page: 508   Topic: Table 12.1: Disorders Discussed in This Chapter That Are Usually First Noticed in Childhood or Adolescence

3. The group session that Dr. Berg held at University Hospital demonstrated that developmental disorders
   a. can all be dealt with.
   b. have similar patterns of development.
   *c. are not always easy to classify.
   d. result from conflict between the parents.

   Pages: 506–507   Topic: Document 12.1: Transcript of the First Meeting of the University Hospital Parent Support Group

4. The major cultural shift that moved children from the realm of "little adults" to a developmental period of their own occurred
   a during the Golden Era of Greece.
   b. in medieval times.
   c. during the Industrial Revolution.
   *d. after the American and French revolutions.

   Page: 508   Topic: Understanding Developmental Psychopathology

5. Researchers studied _____ to help prevent psychological disorders from developing.
   *a. normal children
   b. normal adults
   c. children in mental institutions
   d. disturbed children from "normal" homes

   Page: 508   Topic: Understanding Developmental Psychopathology

6. Three-year-old Solomon wakes up at 7:00 a.m. every morning, eats his breakfast as he quietly chatters with his mother, then shows her what a big boy he is because he can go potty in his "toidy" and doesn't need diapers anymore. Solomon has _____ temperament.
   a. a feisty
   *b. an easy
   c. a slow-to-warm-up
   d. a difficult

   Page: 509   Topic: Temperament and Behavior

7. Four-year-old Joshua does not adapt easily to new situations. His habits are unpredictable, so his parents pretty much let him wake up, eat, and go to sleep when he is ready. They have been having a hard time toilet training him, so they are concerned about whether he will be ready for preschool next year. Joshua has _____ temperament.
   a. an easy
   b. a slow-to-warm-up
   *c. a difficult
   d. a fearful

   Page: 509   Topic: Temperament and Behavior

8. Difficult children are at higher risk than others for developing
   a. ulcers.
   b. depression.
   c. internalizing disorders.
   *d. externalizing disorders.

   Page: 509   Topic: Temperament and Behavior

9. Whether children develop a psychological disorder depends on
   *a. the fit between their temperaments and their environments.
   b. their genetic predisposition.
   c. the type of reinforcement and modeling available in their environment.
   d. how their parents deal with their early socialization.

   Page: 509   Topic: Temperament and Behavior

10. Susanna began walking with support at 12 months, saying simple (although mispronounced) words by 18 months, and was toilet trained by 3 years of age. It appears that Susanna was
    a. advanced in reaching her developmental milestones.
    *b. totally normal in reaching her developmental milestones.
    c. slow in reaching her developmental milestones.
    d. advanced in reaching some developmental milestones, but behind in others.

    Page: 510   Topic: Some Developmental Milestones

11. Matthew's schoolmates don't want to play with him. They say he always smells bad because he can't control his defecation, often eliminating in his pants. Matthew suffers from
    a. poor bladder control.
    b. enuresis.
    *c. encopresis.
    d. endometriosis.

    Page: 510   Topic: Elimination Disorders

12. An important part of growing up to function effectively in society is learning to be
    a. passive.
    b. aggressive.
    c. competitive.
   *d. assertive.

    Page: 511   Topic: Disruptive Behavior and Attention-Deficit Disorders

13. In the case study in the chapter, Paolo's poor school performance was attributed to
   *a. a psychological disturbance.
    b. poor intellectual capacity.
    c. punitive parents.
    d. excessive socializing in class.

    Page: 511   Topic: Document 12.3: School Report on Paolo Armanti

14. Jason, a second grader, often loses his temper, argues with adults, refuses to comply with even the simplest of requests, deliberately annoys his parents and his younger sister (whom he typically blames for his misbehavior), and is usually angry at everyone around him. This pattern has persisted for the past year and has caused him to be suspended from school, to be kicked out of Cub Scouts, and to lose his only friend. Jason's primary diagnosis would be
    a. conduct disorder.
   *b. oppositional defiant disorder.
    c. attention-deficit disorder.
    d. attention-deficit/hyperactivity disorder.

    Page: 512   Topic: Main *DSM-IV* Diagnostic Criteria for Oppositional Defiant Disorder

15. In the case study in the chapter, Dr. Gale administered a battery of tests to Paolo, as well as observing him at home and at school. One of the tests she administered, the Conners Teacher Rating Scale, is designed to
    a. assess intelligence.
    b. determine if a child is living up to his or her potential.
   *c. screen for attentional disorders.
    d. screen for oppositional defiant disorder.

    Page: 512   Topic: Main *DSM-IV* Diagnostic Criteria for Oppositional Defiant Disorder

16. What is the relationship between conduct disorder and antisocial personality disorder?
    a. There is little to no relationship between the two.
    b. They are different names for the same disorder.
    c. If they exist concurrently, *DSM-IV* requires a diagnosis of antisocial personality disorder.
   *d. Conduct disorder is a precursor to antisocial personality disorder.

    Page: 513   Topic: Conduct Disorder

17. Peter has been getting into trouble since he was 7 years old, when he first stole money from his mother's purse. Since then he has been caught lying and stealing too many times to count. Last year, as his sophomore class was holding its honors' ceremony in the high school auditorium, he snuck out and pulled the fire alarm, so everyone had to evacuate the building. Despite showing greater than average irritability and distraction, he has never been violent and is often quite friendly. Peter's diagnosis would be
   *a. moderate conduct disorder, childhood-onset type.
    b. mild conduct disorder, childhood-onset type.
    c. severe conduct disorder, childhood-onset type.
    d. severe conduct disorder, adolescent-onset type.

    Page: 514   Topic: Conduct Disorder

18. Ezekiel is a high school sophomore who lives in the inner city. His father was killed in a drive-by shooting when Ezekiel was 2 years old. Attending the funerals of family and friends has been an unending, lifelong experience for him. For more than 6 years he has exhibited most of the diagnostic characteristics of conduct disorder described in the *DSM-IV*. Ezekiel would
    a. not be diagnosed with conduct disorder because he has been engaging in these behaviors long enough to be diagnosed with antisocial personality disorder.
    *b. not be diagnosed with conduct disorder because his behavior does not violate his age-appropriate societal norms.
    c. be diagnosed with severe conduct disorder, childhood-onset type.
    d. be diagnosed with severe conduct disorder, adolescent-onset type.

    Page: 514   Topic: Conduct Disorder

19. The genetic link for conduct disorder is most likely
    a. an extra Y chromosome.
    b. a missing X chromosome.
    *c. inheritance of a sensation-seeking temperament.
    d. inheritance of an aggressive temperament.

    Page: 515   Topic: Conduct Disorder

20. With respect to the belief that faulty family relationships lead to conduct disorder,
    a. this belief has been supported by the research.
    b. experiments are currently underway to examine such a relationship.
    c. there is little evidence to support such a relationship.
    *d. it may be that the faulty relationships result from the child's disorder.

    Page: 515   Topic: Conduct Disorder

21. What is the relationship between age of onset of conduct disorder and prognosis?
    *a. The prognosis is worse for those whose disorder is first diagnosed in childhood.
    b. The prognosis is worse for those whose disorder is first diagnosed in adolescence.
    c. There is little difference in prognosis in terms of time of onset.
    d. It is not age of onset that is important, but the child's sex—males have a worse prognosis than females.

    Page: 515   Topic: Conduct Disorder

22. In early research on attention-deficit/hyperactivity disorder, Alfred Strauss and his colleagues hypothesized that hyperactivity is
    a. the result of improper parenting.
    *b. a sign that the child is brain damaged.
    c. the result of low cortical stimulation.
    d. a normal behavior, especially in young boys.

    Page: 516   Topic: Attention-Deficit/Hyperactivity Disorder

23. The text notes that the problem with the term *minimally brain damaged* is that
    a. it stigmatizes children who are diagnosed with the disorder.
    b. it provides no insight into how to treat these children.
    *c. children with the diagnosis lack any actual brain damage.
    d. the symptoms overlap other disorders.

    Page: 516   Topic: Attention-Deficit/Hyperactivity Disorder

24. All of the following are diagnostic categories of attention-deficit/hyperactivity disorder EXCEPT
    a. inattention.
    b. hyperactivity.
    c. impulsivity.
   *d. aggression.
   Pages: 516–517   Topic: Attention-Deficit/Hyperactivity Disorder

25. Most children who are diagnosed with attention-deficit/hyperactivity disorder receive the diagnosis after
   *a. an evaluation by their family doctor or pediatrician that takes less than an hour.
    b. an initial evaluation by their family doctor or pediatrician, with a referral to a child psychologist who specializes in diagnosing and treating ADHD.
    c. the school counselor has had extensive interaction with the family and then made a referral to Social Services.
    d. a thorough assessment by a psychologist that includes extensive interviews, behavioral observations, and batteries of psychological tests.
   Page: 516   Topic: Attention-Deficit/Hyperactivity Disorder

26. All of the following are true concerning the prevalence of attention-deficit/hyperactivity disorder EXCEPT:
    a. boys are diagnosed with the disorder much more often than girls.
   *b. there is little difference between boys and girls on measures of hyperactivity.
    c. there is little difference between boys and girls on measures of attention.
    d. differences in diagnosis may reflect a social bias.
   Page: 516   Topic: Attention-Deficit/Hyperactivity Disorder

27. Parents might want their children to be diagnosed with attention-deficit/hyperactivity disorder because
    a. it reduces their own guilt for their children's behavior.
    b. the diagnosis helps them explain why their children are so difficult.
   *c. it may qualify their children for special treatment under the Americans with Disabilities Act.
    d. it may help parents understand their own difficulties as children growing up, because they may have had the disorder without its being diagnosed.
   Page: 517   Topic: Attention-Deficit/Hyperactivity Disorder

28. The MOST common class of drugs for treating attention-deficit/hyperactivity disorder are
    a. tranquilizers.
    b. antidepressants.
    c. antihistamines.
   *d. stimulants.
   Page: 518   Topic: Attention-Deficit/Hyperactivity Disorder

29. Side effects of stimulants for treating attention-deficit/hyperactivity disorder include all of the following EXCEPT
   *a. accelerated growth.
    b. sleeplessness and irritability.
    c. liver damage.
    d. negative self-concept.
   Page: 518   Topic: Attention-Deficit/Hyperactivity Disorder

30. Today most children with attention-deficit/hyperactivity disorder are treated with
    a. stimulants.
    b. cognitive therapy.
    c. behavioral therapy.
    *d. stimulants, cognitive and behavioral therapy, and special education.

    Page: 519   Topic: Attention-Deficit/Hyperactivity Disorder

31. A cognitive-behavioral modification program for treating attention-deficit/hyperactivity disorder would aim at teaching all of the following EXCEPT
    a. monitoring of one's own behavior.
    *b. reinforcment of socially acceptable behavior.
    c. noticing when one's attention is wandering.
    d. engaging in self-talk to keep attention focused.

    Page: 519   Topic: Attention-Deficit/Hyperactivity Disorder

32. Professor Humphrey, a fascinating and brilliant historian, sometimes startles his students by suddenly swearing and barking as he lectures. He also exhibits multiple motor tics, although he is usually able to control both the strange vocalizations and the tics. Professor Humphrey most likely has
    a. Marquise disorder.
    b. Huntington's chorea.
    *c. Tourette's disorder.
    d. Parkinson's disease.

    Page: 519   Topic: Tourette's and Other Tic Disorders

33. The symptom in Tourette's disorder characterized by the shouting of obscenities is called
    a. echolalia.
    b. echopraxia.
    c. copropraxia.
    *d. coprolalia.

    Page: 520   Topic: Tourette's and Other Tic Disorders

34. People with Tourette's disorder would be most likely to have relatives with
    *a. obsessive-compulsive disorder.
    b. depression.
    c. bipolar disorder.
    d. dissociative identity disorder.

    Page: 520   Topic: Tourette's and Other Tic Disorders

35. Children begin to develop strong attachments to their primary caregivers between
    a. birth and 6 months.
    *b. 8 and 12 months.
    c. 12 and 15 months.
    d. 15 months and 2 years.

    Page: 522   Topic: Attachment Formation

36. In Harlow's research with rhesus monkeys, he and his colleagues found that baby monkeys who were raised without their mothers or the presence of other monkeys
    a. learned to adapt to their deprivation.
    b. did not survive to adolescence.
    *c. became profoundly disturbed.
    d. were able to form attachments when they were eventually exposed to other monkeys.

    Page: 523   Topic: Attachment Formation

37. Lupe, a 4-year-old of average intelligence, refuses to be touched or held, and she seems unable to form any strong emotional bonds, especially with her mother. Lupe's mother divorced Lupe's father when it became apparent that he had been physically abusing their daughter. Lupe would be diagnosed with
    a. autism.
    b. childhood schizophrenia.
    c. reactive attachment of the disinhibited subtype.
    *d. reactive attachment of the inhibited subtype.
    Page: 524   Topic: Main *DSM-IV* Criteria for Reactive Attachment Disorder of Infancy or Early Childhood

38. A comparison of Harlow's research with observations of children adopted from European orphanages shows
    *a. as with monkeys, there is a critical period for attachment formation with human children.
    b. as with monkeys, if a human child does not form a close attachment within the first year of life, that child will never be able to form attachments.
    c. unlike monkeys, there is no critical period for attachment formation with human children.
    d. that it is unethical to try to compare rhesus monkeys with human children.
    Pages: 524–525   Topic: Etiology

39. Gracie refuses to go to school because she does not want to leave her mother. Each morning when she wakes up, she tells her mother she has a stomachache or an earache or that her legs won't move, although these ailments disappear when her mother allows her to stay home. Gracie is terrified that if she goes to school, something terrible will happen to her mother while she is gone. Gracie has
    a. obsessive-compulsive disorder.
    *b. separation anxiety disorder.
    c. generalized anxiety disorder.
    d. hypochondriasis.
    Page: 526   Topic: Diagnosis and Etiology

40. Many mental health professionals believe that selective mutism is a type of
    a. autistic behavior.
    b. reactive attachment disorder.
    *c. social phobia.
    d. personality disorder.
    Page: 527   Topic: Diagnosis and Etiology

41. Eloisa has recurring nightmares every evening, usually not long after she falls asleep. They are so frightening that she often screams out, startling her parents, neither of whom can comfort her. The dreams leave her incoherent and terrified and shaking for a long time after she wakes up. However, in the morning she does not remember the dreams. Eloisa has
    a. nightmare disorder.
    b. sleep disorder.
    c. night terror disorder.
    *d. sleep terror disorder.
    Page: 529   Topic: Critical Thinking About . . . 12.1: To Sleep, Perchance to Dream

42. Parasomnias include all of the following EXCEPT
    *a. night tremors.
    b. nightmares.
    c. sleep terrors.
    d. sleepwalking.
    Page: 529   Topic: Critical Thinking About . . . 12.1: To Sleep, Perchance to Dream

43. In the case study in the text about Gordon, the boy who refused to go to school and refused to talk, the most effective therapy was
   a. psychodynamic play therapy.
   *b. cognitive-behavioral self-modeling.
   c. behavioral reinforcement.
   d. use of antidepressants.

   Pages: 528–529   Topic: Treatment

44. How does Asperger's disorder differ from autistic disorder?
   a. Children with Asperger's disorder do not exhibit odd motor behaviors.
   b. Children with Asperger's disorder do not exhibit poor social interaction.
   *c. Children with Asperger's disorder do not exhibit impaired communication.
   d. There are no differences; the two terms are merely different names for the same disorder.

   Page: 531   Topic: Pervasive Developmental Disorders

45. The pervasive developmental disorders include all of the following EXCEPT
   a. autistic disorder.
   b. childhood disintegrative disorder.
   c. Rett's disorder.
   *d. separation anxiety disorder.

   Pages: 530–531   Topic: Pervasive Developmental Disorders

46. Four-year-old Ricky has never been an affectionate child. In fact, when his mother tries to pick him up, he stiffens and arches his back rather than molding to her body and cuddling. Ricky does not speak, nor will he make eye contact with other people. Still sleeping in a crib, Ricky spends hours rocking back and forth, constantly knocking his crib against the apartment wall so that the next door neighbor regularly complains to his mother. Ricky has
   *a. autistic disorder.
   b. Asperger's disorder.
   c. childhood disintegrative disorder.
   d. Rett's disorder.

   Page: 531   Topic: Table 12.11: Main *DSM-IV* Diagnostic Criteria for Autistic Disorder

47. Dustin, an autistic child, parrots what other people say as well as commercial jingles he hears on television ("You deserve a break today"). Dustin is exhibiting
   a. echopraxia.
   *b. echolalia.
   c. copropraxia.
   d. coprolalia.

   Page: 532   Topic: Diagnosis

48. Research with people who have autistic or Asperger's disorder demonstrates that they are unable to
   a. recognize facial features.
   b. respond when spoken to.
   *c. infer mental states.
   d. recognize objects.

   Page: 533   Topic: Diagnosis

49. In those extraordinary cases where a person with a pervasive developmental disorder shows special abilities, such as making complicated mathematical calculations in his or her head, the person has _____ disorder.
   a. autistic
   b. childhood disintegrative
   c. Rett's
   *d. Asperger's
   Page: 534   Topic: Diagnosis

50. Although most of the pervasive developmental disorders mainly affect males, _____ disorder predominately affects females.
   *a. Rett's
   b. autistic
   c. childhood disintegrative
   d. Asperger's
   Page: 534   Topic: Diagnosis

51. Cynthia was a beautiful child when she was born, and she developed normally until she was 2 years old. At that time, she exhibited significant loss of communicative and social skills and a lack of interest in play. She stopped vocalizing and demonstrated stereotypical behaviors, such as waving her hands in front of her eyes for hours on end. Cynthia has
   a. autistic disorder.
   *b. childhood disintegrative disorder.
   c. Asperger's disorder.
   d. Rett's disorder.
   Page: 535   Topic: Table 12.12: Main *DSM-IV* Diagnostic Criteria for Childhood Disintegrative Disorder

52. Which of the following children has the best prognosis?
   a. Armando, who has severe autistic disorder
   b. Constantine, who has childhood disintegrative disorder
   *c. Albert, who has Asperger's disorder
   d. Roland, who has Rett's disorder
   Page: 534   Topic: Epidemiology and Course

53. Psychodynamic therapists suggest that pervasive developmental disorders result from
   a. unresolved unconscious conflicts.
   b. an inability to bond.
   c. repressed sexuality.
   *d. parental behavior.
   Page: 534   Topic: Etiology

54. Which therapeutic paradigm has proved most effective for curing a pervasive developmental disorder?
   a. psychoanalytic
   b. behavioral
   c. biological
   *d. None of them can cure a pervasive developmental disorder.
   Pages: 537–538   Topic: Treatment

55. Jenny suffers from Asperger's disorder. Which combination of treatments will best help her live a higher quality life?
    *a. behavior modification, behaviorally based special education, and speech therapy
    b. behavior modification, drug therapy, and cognitive-behavioral therapy
    c. psychodynamic and drug therapies
    d. behavior modification and facilitated communication

    Page: 538   Topic: Treatment

56. One of the greatest challenges facing the families of children with pervasive developmental disorders when those children grow up is
    a. maintaining relationships with those children.
    *b. making appropriate plans for adulthood.
    c. ensuring the children's autonomy.
    d. providing the least restrictive lifestyle.

    Page: 539   Topic: Treatment

57. Karen felt she was never perfect enough, but she "knew" that if she lost weight, it would help. Despite the expressed concern of her family and friends, she ate only tiny bits of food. She advised those who scolded her that she kept healthy by exercising, which she did to excess. She became so thin that she stopped menstruating, yet she intensely feared becoming fat. In fact, she believed she was fat. Karen, who ultimately died, had
    a. bulimia nervosa.
    *b. anorexia nervosa.
    c. binge-eating disorder.
    d. body dysmorphic disorder.

    Page: 540   Topic: Feeding and Eating Disorders

58. Which eating disorder is currently being evaluated for possible inclusion in the *DSM?*
    a. anorexia nervosa
    b. bulimia nervosa
    *c. binge-eating
    d. binge-eating/purging

    Page: 541   Topic: Feeding and Eating Disorders

59. Brandon's mother often feels she should physically restrain her boy for his own well-being. Since he was an infant, Brandon has seemed to crave dirt, sand, and other gritty substances that have no nutritive value. Brandon has
    a. rumination disorder.
    b. feeding disorder.
    *c. pica.
    d. anorexia.

    Page: 542   Topic: Feeding and Eating Disorders

60. With respect to the potential complications of eating disorders,
    a. pica may produce high blood pressure.
    b. binge-eating may cause poisoning.
    c. binge-eating may cause tooth decay.
    *d. anorexia may cause death.

    Page: 543   Topic: Prevalence and Course

61. All of the following Axis I disorders are commonly found among people with anorexia and bulimia EXCEPT
   *a. bipolar disorder.
   b. depression.
   c. obsessive-compulsive disorder.
   d. substance abuse disorders.

   Page: 544   Topic: Etiology

62. With respect to the etiology of eating disorders, the text supports which approach?
   *a. the social-psychological theory, which focuses on cultural standards of beauty
   b. the psychodynamic view, which says that eating disorders are symbolic representations of unconscious conflicts
   c. the behavioral approach, which presumes that food avoidance or overindulgence is somehow reinforced
   d. the family systems approach, which claims that families with eating-disordered members are enmeshed

   Pages: 544–545   Topic: Etiology

63. The first goal of any treatment for anorexia nervosa is to
   a. help the client to understand the cause of the disorder.
   *b. help the client to gain enough weight to overcome immediate health threats.
   c. teach the client effective self-monitoring skills.
   d. get the family involved in monitoring the client's eating habits.

   Page: 547   Topic: Treatment

64. Which of the following have studies evaluating prevention of eating disorders on college campuses found?
   a. Students who are exposed to health and nutrition information through dissemination of literature are less concerned about weight than are those not exposed.
   b. Students who are exposed to health and nutrition information in class lectures are less concerned about weight than are those not exposed.
   *c. Students who are exposed to health and nutrition information in dining halls are less concerned about weight than are those not exposed.
   d. None of the campaigns to counter eating disorders have been effective.

   Page: 548   Topic: Prevention

65. Secondary prevention for groups at high risk for eating disorders has focused mainly on
   a. sororities.
   b. students seeking help in the counseling centers.
   c. high achievers.
   *d. athletes.

   Page: 548   Topic: Prevention

TRUE-FALSE QUESTIONS

66. Frustration and marital conflict are the primary underlying causes of developmental disorders. (F)

   Page: 508   Topic: Understanding Developmental Psychopathology

67. Despite their different emphases, all psychological paradigms agree that elimination disorders are most likely to occur when toilet training is harsh or inconsistent. (T)

   Pages: 509–510   Topic: Elimination Disorders

68. Adoption and twin studies have confirmed a genetic link for conduct disorder. (T)

   Page: 515   Topic: Conduct Disorder

69. Learning disorders lead to conduct disorder in young children. (F)

    Page: 515   Topic: Conduct Disorder

70. There are large regional differences in the prevalence of attention-deficit/hyperactivity disorder. (T)

    Page: 516   Topic: Attention-Deficit/Hyperactivity Disorder

71. Too much sugar in the diet has been found to be one of the causes of the hyperactive behavior of children with attention-deficit/hyperactivity disorder. (F)

    Page: 518   Topic: Attention-Deficit/Hyperactivity Disorder

72. Stimulants have a paradoxical calming effect in children with attention-deficit/hyperactivity disorder. (F)

    Page: 518   Topic: Attention-Deficit/Hyperactivity Disorder

73. The criteria for diagnosing Tourette's disorder have not changed from its original description. (T)

    Pages: 519–520   Topic: Tourette's and Other Tic Disorders

74. In replicating Harlow's monkey studies with humans, researchers have found very similar results. (F)

    Page: 523   Topic: Attachment Formation

75. Studies of children adopted from European orphanages have found that the older children are when they are adopted, the more likely they are to develop an attachment disorder. (T)

    Page: 524   Topic: Etiology

76. Pervasive developmental disorders are the most serious psychopathological conditions occurring in childhood. (T)

    Page: 530   Topic: Pervasive Developmental Disorders

77. Despite their social and communication handicaps, most people with pervasive developmental disorders display great cognitive abilities in other areas. (F)

    Page: 534   Topic: Diagnosis

78. The story about Temple Grandin, an animal behaviorist who has a pervasive developmental disorder, demonstrates that people with these disorders can go on to lead normal lives. (F)

    Page: 536   Topic: Highlight 12.2: Thinking Like an Animal

79. To date, the most effective therapy found for treating pervasive childhood disorders is facilitated communication. (F)

    Pages: 538–539   Topic: Treatment

80. The hallmark of bulimia is binge-eating. (T)

    Page: 540   Topic: Feeding and Eating Disorders

81. With respect to anorexia nervosa, the sex ratio of 9 females to 1 male has not changed for decades. (T)

    Page: 542   Topic: Prevalence and Course

82. The single technique that those with anorexia use to lose weight is to go on starvation diets. (F)

    Page: 544   Topic: Etiology

83. Antidepressant drugs have not been highly effective in treating anorexia. (T)

    Page: 547   Topic: Etiology

84. Health insurers are proactive in providing the necessary hospital care for people with eating disorders. (F)

Page: 546   Topic: Highlight 12.3: Starved Out

85. Studies have found that college students who are exposed to health and nutrition information in dining halls are less concerned about weight than are those who are not exposed. (T)

Page: 548   Topic: Prevention

SHORT-ANSWER QUESTIONS

86. Explain the three characteristic temperaments described by Chess and Alexander (1995).

Easy children have regular patterns of elimination, eating, and sleeping; they adapt readily to new environments; and even when they are distressed, their emotional reactions are usually mild. Slow-to-warm-up children take longer to adapt to new situations than do easy children, but they eventually adjust; their emotional reactions are mild. Difficult children have irregular patterns of eating, sleeping, and elimination; they are slow to adapt to new situations; and they have intense, usually negative, emotional reactions (such as tantrums).

Page: 509   Topic: Temperament and Behavior

87. Explain the etiological theory that suggests a sensation-seeking temperament as the genetic mechanism for conduct disorder.

The idea is that people with conduct disorder are chronically underaroused. To make up for this, they are always seeking excitement. When their environment lacks socially acceptable opportunities for excitement, they turn to antisocial behaviors.

Page: 515   Topic: Conduct Disorder

88. Discuss the problems with the *DSM-IV* diagnostic criteria for attention-deficit/hyperactivity disorder.

Norms are unavailable for many attentional behaviors, and behavior depends on context. Thus parents, teachers, and clinicians often fail to agree about which children suffer from ADHD. Diagnostic unreliability may explain the large regional differences in the prevalence of ADHD.

Pages: 516–518   Topic: Attention-Deficit/Hyperactivity Disorder

89. Discuss the evidence that supports a neurochemical basis for Tourette's disorder.

The discovery that small doses of haloperidol, a dopamine-suppressing drug used to treat schizophrenia, suppress Tourette's symptoms in many people has led to the hypothesis that Tourette's patients may have an excess of dopamine. Further evidence for this hypothesis comes from the finding that drugs that increase dopamine levels, such as L-dopa, which is used in Parkinson's disease, tend to increase the severity of tics.

Pages: 520–521   Topic: Tourette's and Other Tic Disorders

90. Describe the various treatments used for reactive attachment disorder.

Holding therapy requires parents to initiate physical contact with their child, by force if necessary, with the idea that contact is required to "break through" to children who "freeze out" their parents; advocates of holding therapy say its safe application requires professional training ($7,000 per course), but many psychologists are skeptical about its rationale and efficacy. More typically, multiple treatment modalities are used, including role playing, modeling, and teaching social interaction skills. Family members are counseled to identify impediments to attachment formation and to learn how to reinforce appropriate behavior. Typically, primary caregivers require individual therapy to deal with their feelings of guilt, inadequacy, and secondary depression. Abusive parents require treatment for anger control. Support groups help parents in many ways, such as in finding respite care and in learning about treatment options.

Pages: 525–526   Topic: Treatment

91. Discuss possible causes of and factors that maintain separation anxiety disorder.

A child may have experienced separation from the parents, through death or divorce. In other cases, it may arise from overprotectiveness, when parents worry excessively about harm coming to their child if the chid is outside their immediate purview, and they communicate their anxiety to the child, who then learns to fear separation. Sometimes the parents themselves have the disorder. Staying home is reinforcing for the child because it reduces anxiety and offers secondary rewards, such as maternal attention.

Page: 526   Topic: Diagnosis and Etiology

92. Describe the various sleep disorders that can affect children.

Parasomnias include (1) nightmare disorder: when nightmares are so frequent that they cause clinical distress or impair a person's functioning. (2) Sleep terror disorder: after awakening from a nightmare, children remain incoherent and terrified for a prolonged period; the nightmares occur during the first hour or two of sleep, the child's heart races, breathing is shallow, and the child is covered in sweat; some children run around the room in a frenzy; they may not recognize their parents and are not easily comforted, but after the 15- to 30-minute episode, they sleep peacefully, with no memory of the dream the next morning. (3) Sleepwalking disorder: occurs early in sleep; sleepwalkers move around their room (or even further), but do not recognize or respond to others; they have no memory of the episode the next day. Dyssomnias are disturbances in the amount, quality, or timing of sleep.

Page: 529   Topic: Critical Thinking About . . . 12.1: To Sleep, Perchance to Dream

93. Describe the procedure called self-modeling, which was used in the case study about Gordon, the boy who refused to talk.

The therapist had Gordon's parents tape-record him answering questions posed by his mother; the clinician then taped his teacher asking the same questions and edited the two tapes so it appeared that Gordon was responding to the teacher's questions. She repeatedly played the tape for Gordon and rewarded him with praise and toys during the segments in which he "answered" the teacher's questions. After many sessions, this procedure induced Gordon to say a few words to the therapist. She then added more people to the tape so that Gordon could hear himself "answering" questions posed by various adults and children.

Pages: 529–530   Topic: Treatment

94. Describe the characteristics of autistic disorder and Asperger's disorder, and explain how they differ.

Autism is marked by poor social interactions, impaired communication, and odd motor behaviors. Asperger's disorder is similar to autistic disorder, but without the serious language and communication problems.

Pages: 530–531   Topic: Pervasive Developmental Disorders

95. Describe the "theory of mind" focus as it applies to autism.

Interpersonal functioning requires the ability to assign mental states to oneself and others. To know whether to laugh with or console another person, we must be able to infer whether that person is happy or sad, which requires an understanding that other people have mental states containing feelings, wishes, and desires. This understanding is apparent in normal 2-year-olds, but it is missing in people with autistic disorder. People with autistic and Asperger's disorders are unable to see the world from another person's point of view.

Pages: 531–534   Topic: Diagnosis

96. What have the researchers concluded about the etiology of pervasive developmental disorders?

After enlisting every conceivable blood test, hormonal assay, neuropsychological test, and imaging technique, and evaluating twin studies, there is no agreement on the neurological defects that cause the symptoms and signs of pervasive disorders. All that can presently be concluded is that people with autism and Asperger's disorder probably have a congenital vulnerability that combines with a trigger (a virus, a toxin, birth trauma) resulting in an inability to form normal human attachments and, in people with autism, a language disability as well. In childhood disintegrative disorder and Rett's disorder, the trigger occurs later in childhood, and mental retardation is almost always severe. There are no clear-cut biochemical, genetic, or neurological markers unique to any of the pervasive developmental disorders.

Page: 537   Topic: Etiology

97. Explain the process and purpose of facilitated communication, as well as the controversy concerning it.

Based on the notion that there is a person trapped inside the person with a pervasive developmental disorder, a "facilitator" is employed to "help" the child communicate by using a computer. The facilitator gently holds the child's hand over the keyboard, and the child types out what he or she wants to say. However, facilitators typically have only a day or two of "training," and it is likely that the thoughts being communicated are the facilitator's, not the person's being facilitated. The problems of people with pervasive disorders are so great and the desire to help them so intense that parents—and even some professionals— allow their hopes to overwhelm the evidence that this process does not work.

Pages: 538–539   Topic: Treatment

98. Differentiate between anorexia nervosa and bulimia nervosa.

The essential features of anorexia nervosa are that the individual refuses to maintain a minimally normal body weight, is intensely afraid of gaining weight, and exhibits a significant disturbance in the perception of the shape or size of his or her body; in addition, postmenarcheal females with this disorder are amenorrheic. In the restricting subtype of anorexia, weight loss is accomplished primarily through dieting, fasting, or excessive exercise, not through regular binge-eating and purging; in the binge-eating/purging subtype, during the episode the individual will binge-eat and then purge through self-induced vomiting or the misuse of laxatives, diuretics, or enemas. The essential features of bulimia nervosa are binge-eating and inappropriate compensatory methods to prevent weight gain (e.g., self-induced vomiting); the individual's self-evaluation is also excessively influenced by body shape and weight. Individuals whose binge-eating behavior occurs only during anorexia nervosa are given the diagnosis "anorexia nervosa, binge-eating/ purging type."

Page: 540   Topic: Feeding and Eating Disorders

99. Describe the eating disorder pica and explain the part that culture plays in diagnosis.

Pica, which is most often found among young children and pregnant women, is a disorder in which the person will eat practically anything that is nonnutritive (e.g., dirt, laundry starch, chalk, buttons, paper, cigarette butts, matches, sand, soap, toothpaste, etc.), and this behavior is inappropriate to developmental level. However, cultural practices must be considered when making the diagnosis because members of cultures that sanction the consumption of odd substances (e.g., clay) are not suffering from a psychological disorder.

Page: 542   Topic: Feeding and Eating Disorders

100. What is the dilemma of getting health care for people with anorexia?

Hospital care is a necessity for people whose weight loss puts them in danger of death. Yet managed care organizations and health insurers provide only meager benefits for the inpatient treatment of eating disorders. Many people who need treatment are priced out. It is ironic that the psychological disorder with the highest mortality rate (about 10% of those with anorexia nervosa will die of their disorder) is one that insurance companies refuse to cover.

Page: 542   Topic: Highlight 12.3: Starved Out

ESSAY QUESTIONS

101. One of your friends, a medical student, has told you she wants to become a psychiatrist. More specifically, she is fascinated with the "mental diseases" of children and teens. When you ask her about the courses she'll be taking, you notice that she does not mention developmental psychology. How would you explain to her that learning about developmental psychology will help her understand the psychological disorders of children and adolescents.

    Discuss the relationship between temperament and behavior, as well as developmental milestones, and the theories behind the various disorders of childhood and adolescence that relate to the child's development.

102. You've just taken your little cousin to the zoo, and she became extremely upset because she noticed one little monkey was off in a cage all by himself, and he looked very sad. She asks you why you think the monkey was alone and what will happen to the monkey if he never gets to be with other monkeys, especially his mother. Then she asks you if people act the same way as monkeys. What could you tell her about attachment, why it is psychologically and biologically necessary for monkeys and human children to form attachments, and what happens when the attachment process goes awry?

    Discuss the importance of attachment in healthy biological and psychological development, look at normal separation anxiety, then address attachment and separation anxiety disorders.

103. Knowing that you are interested in childhood psychopathology and that you are taking this class in abnormal psychology, the secretary of your local religious congregation asks you to address the parents of some children who have been diagnosed with a variety of childhood disorders. She asks that you address the main psychological disorders that are first observed in childhood and adolescence, what might cause these disorders, how they are generally treated, and the effects of the disorders on other family members. What could you tell your audience?

    Discuss the various disorders (disruptive behavior, attention-deficit hyperactivity, Tourette's, attachment and separation anxiety, pervasive developmental, and feeding and eating disorders), possible etiological factors, different forms of treatment and their degree of effectiveness, and the effects of these disorders on the family.

104. Over lunch one day, you and your friends get into a discussion of the eating disorders. One of your friends says, "You know who I think has an eating disorder? Calista Flockhart on *Ally McBeal,* even though she says she doesn't!" Another friend says, "Yeah, well, you know who really *did* have an eating disorder and it wound up killing her—Karen Carpenter, the singer." The discussion heats up about what causes eating disorders, who may or may not have one, and how you can tell. Knowing you're studying just this very topic, your friends turn to you and ask you about the eating disorders—what causes them and how they can be treated. Most important, they want to know how they can be prevented. What knowledge could you share with them?

    Discuss the diagnoses of the various eating disorders, particularly differentiating between the two subtypes of anorexia and bulimia; then discuss etiology, treatment—dismal as the prognosis may be—and prevention strategies.

105. You have been invited to talk to a group of parents at your local youth center. They are concerned about the apparent increase in childhood disorders and want you to help them plan an intervention program. The program is to address the needs of children already diagnosed with a disorder as well as strategies to prevent these disorders from developing in the first place. Explain the processes, techniques, and strategies you would suggest to these concerned parents.

    Address the various types of treatment for the different disorders, as well as primary, secondary, and tertiary prevention strategies, indicating how effective each might be.

CHAPTER 13
SEXUAL AND RELATED PROBLEMS OF ADULT LIFE

MULTIPLE-CHOICE QUESTIONS

1. Sexual activity with a prepubescent child is referred to as
   *a. pedophilia.
   b. pedophobia.
   c. paraphilia.
   d. paraphobia.

   Page: 556   Topic: The Predator

2. From a clinical point of view, pedophilia is a
   a. crime.
   *b. psychological disorder.
   c. treatable disorder.
   d. sin.

   Page: 556   Topic: The Predator

3. In the case study in the text, Peter Hall's disorder was one of the paraphilias, which are defined as
   a. sexual activity with young children and adolescents.
   b. difficulties in performing sexual acts.
   *c. unusual, harmful, or unacceptable sexual desires and acts.
   d. discomfort with one's assigned sex role.

   Page: 556   Topic: The Predator

4. During most of the medieval period,
   a   sex was considered holy and enjoyable.
   b. engaging in sex was particularly holy on the Sabbath.
   c. sex was a taboo topic.
   *d. care was taken to protect men from seductive witches.

   Page: 556   Topic: Paraphilias

5. Sex became a taboo topic
   *a. during the reign of Britain's Queen Victoria.
   b. in the Middle Ages.
   c. during the era of the Holy Roman Empire.
   d. during the Golden Age of Greece.

   Page: 556   Topic: Paraphilias

6. How did von Krafft-Ebing preserve his reputation while writing explicitly about sex?
   a. He wrote in medical terms.
   *b. His descriptions of the various sex acts were written in Latin.
   c. His descriptions of the various sex acts were poetic and circumscribed.
   d. He wrote in biblical terms.

   Page: 557   Topic: Paraphilias

7. Von Krafft-Ebing was a supporter of all of the following EXCEPT
   a. homosexual law reform.
   b. treatment rather than punishment for people with paraphilias.
   *c. masturbation.
   d. liberalizing attitudes toward sex.

   Page: 557   Topic: Paraphilias

8. In his research on sexual behavior, Kinsey found
   a. that masturbation was common among men, but rare among women.
   b. little variation in the sexual practices of Americans.
   c. that his respondents were reluctant to discuss their sexual experiences.
   *d. that homosexual experiences were reported by people who were mainly heterosexual.

   Page: 558   Topic: Paraphilias

9. The text's author attributes today's more liberal attitude toward sex to
   *a. the sexual revolution of the 1960s.
   b. a rebellion against the Victorian era of sexual repression.
   c. increased knowledge and information.
   d. the increasing cultural diversity of our society.

   Page: 558   Topic: Paraphilias

10. The sex practices that continue to be considered unacceptable today
    a. will probably become more acceptable in the future.
    *b. cause suffering to the individual who engages in them or to other people.
    c. are the same practices that have traditionally been unacceptable.
    d. are genetically based.

    Page: 558   Topic: Paraphilias

11. Eroica is a junior in college. If her sexual experiences are similar to those of other university-age women, the sexual experience in which she MOST engages would be
    a. masturbating alone.
    b. sexual intercourse.
    *c. kissing on the lips.
    d. deep kissing.

    Page: 559   Topic: Table 13.1: Sexual Experiences of University-Age Women

12. Arden is getting serious about the woman he has been dating and would like to have sexual intercourse with her. However, he is concerned about sexually transmitted diseases. What should he do?
    a. He should assume that she is more concerned than he is, so she will undoubtedly be prepared with a female condom.
    b. He should avoid embarrassment by not bringing up the topic of safe sex.
    c. He should either break up with her to avoid the temptation of having sex or marry her so they will be sure to be in a monogamous relationship.
    *d. He should introduce the topic of safe sex and reassure her that he enjoys being with her but that they need to discuss the topic before engaging in sex.

    Page: 558   Topic: Highlight 13.1: How to Be Smart About Sex

13. According to the *DSM-IV*, the paraphilias are characterized by all of the following intense sexual fantasies EXCEPT
   *a. sex by oneself.
   b. sex with nonhuman objects.
   c. sex that involves suffering.
   d. sex with children.

   Page: 558   Topic: Diagnosis

14. The most frequently searched Internet topic is:
   a. scientific information.
   *b. sex.
   c. erotica.
   d. music.

   Page: 560   Topic: Highlight 13.2: Surfing for Sex

15. All paraphilias share the central characteristic of sexual behavior that
   a. disturbs other people.
   b. involves a loving, consensual relationship with young children.
   *c. is disconnected from a loving, consensual relationship with another adult.
   d. involves a fascination with the personal objects of someone of the opposite sex.

   Page: 560   Topic: Diagnosis

16. Mitchell exposes his genitals to strangers, fantasizing that these strangers will find the display sexually arousing. This type of paraphilia is classified in the *DSM-IV* as
   a. flashing.
   b. fetishism.
   c. voyeurism.
   *d. exhibitionism.

   Page: 560   Topic: Exhibitionism

17. Robert always has young boys around his house. He entertains them with stories of his life on the stage and in the movies, most of which were made long before they were born. He enjoys fondling these boys and engaging in sexual intercourse with them. Robert is a
   *a. pedophile.
   b. frotteurist.
   c. voyeur.
   d. exhibitionist.

   Page: 561   Topic: Pedophilia

18. All of the following are characteristic of transvestic fetishism EXCEPT that it
   a. begins in childhood or adolescence.
   *b. is done by homosexual males to entertain an audience.
   c. involves males wearing female clothes.
   d. may progress from wearing one article of female clothing to entire outfits and makeup.

   Page: 562   Topic: Transvestic Fetishism

19. Rape involves all of the following EXCEPT
   a. sexual penetration.
   b. menace or force.
   *c. a sexual act.
   d. lack of consent.

   Page: 562   Topic: Highlight 13.3: Rape Is Not Sex

20. The prevalence of paraphilias is difficult to know because
    a. most paraphiliacs are in jail and are therefore difficult to survey.
    b. most paraphiliacs lie about their activities on surveys or in interviews.
    c. paraphiliacs typically perform their activities in their own homes, so they go unnoticed.
    *d. paraphiliacs rarely seek clinical assistance.

    Page: 563   Topic: Paraphilias Not Otherwise Specified

21. Statutory rape
    *a. is punishable by a prison sentence.
    b. is a psychological disorder.
    c. involves an unwilling partner.
    d. infers that the "perpetrator" is at least 5 years older than the "victim."

    Page: 565   Topic: Critical Thinking About . . . 13.1: Sex Crimes and Misdemeanors

22. Peter Hall, from the case study in the text,
    a. understood that having sex with the boys in his care might be expected to harm them psychologically.
    *b. believed that he had not harmed the boys he had sex with.
    c. knew that the boys did not want to have sex with him but did not feel he had caused them any harm.
    d. accused the boys in his care of sexually molesting him.

    Page: 564   Topic: Document 13.3: Excerpts from Peter Hall's Court-Ordered Psychological Evaluation

23. The psychological evaluation of Peter Hall (case study in the text) suggested that his pattern of scores on the MMPI-2 were consistent with which Axis II diagnosis?
    a. mental retardation
    b. conduct disorder
    *c. antisocial personality disorder
    d. borderline personality disorder

    Page: 566   Topic: Document 13.3: Excerpts from Peter Hall's Court-Ordered Psychological Evaluation

24. Which of the following would NOT be considered "normal" in terms of *DSM-IV* classifications of sexual disorders?
    a. Cynthia, who uses a penis-shaped vibrator to masturbate.
    b. Clifford, who has sex with an inflatable rubber doll designed for masturbation.
    c. Cornell, who masturbates while watching pornographic videos alone in his home.
    *d. Carl, who uses women's underwear to masturbate.

    Page: 566   Topic: Cultural Influences on Diagnosis

25. A major problem in determining biological causes of the paraphilias is
    *a. small sample size.
    b. inability to measure hormone levels at the time of the paraphiliac acts.
    c. ethical restrictions on increasing hormone levels to evaluate their contribution.
    d. lack of female comparison groups.

    Page: 567   Topic: Biological Causes

26. All of the following are possible psychosocial causes of paraphilias EXCEPT
    a. childhood and adolescent experiences that limit the person's ability to be aroused by consensual sexual activity.
    *b. extraordinarily high levels of male sex hormones.
    c. environments that foster repressive, guilt-producing attitudes toward sex.
    d. having been sexually abused as a child.

    Page: 567   Topic: Biological Causes

27. According to the psychodynamic explanations of paraphiliac behavior, someone who seeks physical punishment and humiliation during sex may be
   a. seeking a way out of responsibilities.
   b. overcoming feelings of inadequacy.
   *c. displaying guilt about sexual urges.
   d. passively seeking a position of power.

   Page: 568   Topic: Social and Psychological Causes

28. Most treatments for the paraphilias have been aimed at
   a. exhibitionists.
   b. fetishists.
   c. sexual masochists.
   *d. pedophiles.

   Page: 569   Topic: Treatment and Prevention

29. Which treatment has been the MOST successful for pedophilia?
   *a. cognitive-behavioral
   b. aversive conditioning
   c. castration
   d. psychodynamic

   Page: 569   Topic: Treatment and Prevention

30. A technique used by behavioral therapists that attempts to reorient the client's fantasies to a more "normal" experience is
   a. phallometric testing.
   *b. masturbatory reconditioning.
   c. chemical castration.
   d. cingulotomy.

   Page: 569   Topic: Treatment and Prevention

31. Primary prevention efforts for the paraphilias have been aimed at
   a. early sex education in schools.
   b. intervention through religious institutions.
   *c. censoring paraphiliac pornography.
   d. heavy jail sentences for offenders.

   Page: 570   Topic: Treatment and Prevention

32. Megan's Law requires
   a. school programs to encourage children to report suspicious people or incidents.
   b. civil commitment of sexual predators who are about to be released from prison.
   c. forced castration of sexual predators.
   *d. police registration of sex offenders and informing communities of their presence.

   Page: 570   Topic: Treatment and Prevention

33. The most common sleep disorder, _____ , is difficulty in initiating or maintaining sleep or having sleep that is not perceived as restful.
   *a. primary insomnia
   b. narcolepsy
   c. hypersomnia
   d. circadian-rhythm sleep disorder

   Page: 571   Topic: Highlight 13.4: Sleep Disorders

34. Marcia has irresistible "sleep attacks" in which she simply falls asleep at her desk in her law office, while driving, or even when she is in court. Marcia has
    a. primary insomnia
    *b. narcolepsy
    c. hypersomnia
    d. circadian-rhythm sleep disorder

    Page: 571   Topic: Highlight 13.4: Sleep Disorders

35. In the case study, as a result of his sexual abuse by Peter Hall, Jared
    a. became a sexual predator.
    b. was unable to date women.
    *c. was unable to have sexual relations with a woman.
    d. became homosexual.

    Page: 572   Topic: The Prey

36. William H. Masters and Virginia E. Johnson followed up Kinsey's research by
    a. more intensive surveys of people's sexual behavior.
    b. in-depth interviews assessing people's sexual behavior.
    c. correlational studies of sexual practices and sexual disorders.
    *d. direct observations of people's sexual behavior under controlled laboratory conditions.

    Page: 573   Topic: Human Sexual Response

37. Masters and Johnson set out to
    *a. describe how physical and psychological mechanisms work together to control sexual responsiveness.
    b. determine which sexual behaviors lead to sexual dysfunction.
    c. develop an effective treatment for the paraphilias.
    d. describe the sexual patterns of heterosexual and homosexual males and females in the United States.

    Page: 573   Topic: Human Sexual Response

38. With respect to hormonal secretions, normally
    a. females have both androgens and estrogens; males have only androgens.
    *b. females and males both have androgens and estrogens.
    c. females have only estrogens; males have both androgens and estrogens.
    d. females have only estrogens; males have only androgens.

    Page: 573   Topic: Human Sexual Response

39. Which period of the sexual response cycle is experienced only by men?
    a. desire
    b. excitement
    *c. refractory
    d. plateau

    Page: 576   Topic: Table 13.3: Five Phases of the Sexual Response Cycle

40. The National Health and Social Life Survey found that during the preceding year
    a. equally as many males as females claimed to always have an orgasm while having sex with their partner.
    b. for females, but not for males, sexual satisfaction is directly tied to having an orgasm.
    c. the males were surprisingly accurate in reporting how often their female partners experienced orgasm.
    *d. females did not need to have an orgasm to be physically and emotionally satisfied with sex.

    Page: 577   Topic: Highlight 13.5: Sex and the Big "O"

41. Disorders of sexual desire affect the _____ phase of the sexual response cycle.
    *a. desire
    b. excitement
    c. plateau
    d. orgasmic

    Page: 576   Topic: Human Sexual Response

42. Harry is unable to develop or maintain an adequate erection long enough to complete sexual activity. He has
    a. hypoactive sexual desire disorder.
    *b. male erectile disorder.
    c. male orgasmic disorder
    d. premature ejaculation.

    Page: 578   Topic: Table 13.4: *DSM-IV* Sexual Dysfunctions

43. Sally consistently either has a delay in reaching orgasm or is unable to achieve orgasm following normal sexual excitement. She has
    a. female sexual arousal disorder.
    b. sexual aversion disorder.
    *c. female orgasmic disorder.
    d. vaginismus.

    Page: 578   Topic: Table 13.4: *DSM-IV* Sexual Dysfunctions

44. _____ is the complex set of feelings, cognitions, and fantasies that motivate people to engage in sex.
    a. Lust
    b. Love
    c. Duty
    *d. Desire

    Page: 577   Topic: Sexual Desire Disorders

45. Augusta has never had much interest in any type of real or fantasy sex, and this lack of interest seems to have negatively affected her life. Augusta has which type of sexual dysfunction?
    *a. hypoactive sexual desire disorder
    b. hyperactive sexual desire disorder
    c. sexual aversion disorder
    d. female sexual arousal disorder

    Pages: 577–578   Topic: Sexual Desire Disorders

46. Which of the following is NOT contained in the *DSM-IV?*
    a. hypoactive sexual desire disorder
    *b. hyperactive sexual desire disorder
    c. sexual aversion disorder
    d. female sexual arousal disorder

    Page: 578   Topic: Sexual Desire Disorders

47. The *DSM-IV* considers compulsive sexual behavior
    a. a form of obsessive-compulsive disorder.
    b. hyperactive sexual desire disorder.
    *c. a sign of some other disorder.
    d. a form of healthy behavior.

    Page: 580   Topic: Highlight 13.6: Addicted to Sex

48. Although Faith engaged in hugging and kissing, she actively avoided any other type of sexual activity. She was able to find a husband who was satisfied with the limits on their sex life. According to the *DSM-IV*, Faith would
   a. be diagnosed with sexual aversion disorder.
   b. be diagnosed with hypoactive sexual desire disorder.
   c. be diagnosed with sexual phobia.
   *d. not be diagnosed with a disorder.

   Page: 579   Topic: Sexual Desire Disorders

49. With respect to the sexual arousal disorders, the text notes that
   *a. the *DSM-IV*'s concentration on genital lubrication as a causative factor in female sexual arousal disorder is misleading.
   b. arousal disorders develop after the individual has become sexually active.
   c. the common underlying factor that causes women to report a lack of arousal is a lack of genital lubrication.
   d. the same physiological factors are responsible for lack of arousal in men and in women.

   Page: 579   Topic: Sexual Arousal Disorders

50. The most common reason for men to visit clinics for help with a sexual dysfunction is
   a. sexual aversion disorder.
   *b. erectile dysfunction.
   c. male orgasmic disorder.
   d. premature ejaculation.

   Page: 579   Topic: Sexual Arousal Disorders

51. What percentage of women never experience an orgasm?
   a. less than 5%
   b. 5–10%
   *c. 10–15%
   d. 15–20%

   Page: 581   Topic: Orgasmic Disorders

52. Which of the following women has female orgasmic disorder?
   a. Vanessa, who is not concerned about the fact that she has never had an orgasm
   b. Valerie, whose husband rushes through foreplay and does not know how to stimulate her to reach orgasm
   c. Victoria, who can achieve orgasm only through oral stimulation, which is her favorite type of sexual activity
   *d. Veronica, whose frustration over not reaching orgasm is having a negative effect on her marriage

   Page: 581   Topic: Orgasmic Disorders

53. Who is most likely to experience premature ejaculation?
   *a. Seventeen-year-old Roland, who is afraid his lover's husband will come home any minute.
   b. Forty-year-old Robert, who is separated from his wife and enjoying the company of another woman.
   c. Twenty-five-year-old Raymond, who is trying to impregnate his wife so that they can have the child they both want.
   d. Sixty-five-year-old Russell, who, together with his wife of 40 years, is trying various new positions from the *Kama Sutra*.

   Page: 581   Topic: Orgasmic Disorders

54. Dyspareunia is diagnosed when
    a. pain during sex is the result of a physiological condition.
    *b. pain during sex has a strong psychological component.
    c. involuntary contractions of the perineal muscles around the vagina prohibit intercourse.
    d. a woman consistently reaches orgasm before her partner.

    Page: 581   Topic: Sexual Pain Disorders

55. With respect to prevalence of sexual dysfunctions,
    a. African American women are more likely to report being satisfied with their sex life than are White women.
    b. single people report fewer sexual dysfunctions than married people.
    *c. married people report fewer sexual dysfunctions than single people.
    d. a married person in ill health is more likely to have a sexual dysfunction than a healthy single person.

    Page: 582   Topic: Epidemiology and Course

56. John is getting on in years and his testosterone levels are gradually decreasing, leading to fewer spontaneous sexual fantasies. In terms of his sex life,
    a. John will gradually lose all interest in sex.
    b. testosterone levels cannot predict sexual desire.
    c. John may make up for the decrease by getting estrogen shots.
    *d. John may make up for the decrease by watching erotic films or engaging in extended foreplay.

    Page: 582   Topic: Etiology

57. A month ago, Trevor lost his job. He and his wife had bought a new house a year ago and have a huge monthly payment. They are worried about losing their house and their savings. Recently Trevor has been unable to get an erection when he and his wife have attempted intercourse. This is something that has never happened to him before. The proper diagnosis is
    *a. adjustment disorder.
    b. anxiety disorder.
    c. transitory erectile disorder.
    d. erectile disorder.

    Page: 583   Topic: Etiology

58. One of the major problems of erectile disorder is that it can create
    a. penile infection.
    *b. a vicious cycle that creates anxiety and increased chances of erectile failure.
    c. other sexual dysfunctions.
    d. atrophy of the testicles.

    Page: 583   Topic: Etiology

59. Which treatment would a woman with vaginismus MOST likely use?
    a. hormone replacement therapy
    b. vaginal lubricants
    *c. increasingly larger metal rods
    d. a sex surrogate

    Page: 584   Topic: Treatment

60. As a result of war injuries and getting on in years, Robert has been experiencing erectile disorder. His wife, Elizabeth, has tried a variety of strategies, including sexy negligees, but none of these strategies have worked. Robert and Elizabeth both have the desire. The most likely treatment for Robert is
   a. a penile pump implant.
   b. injectable drugs.
   c. nitrate medications.
   *d. Viagra.

   Page: 584   Topic: Treatment

61. All of the following treatment techniques are used in modern sex therapy EXCEPT
   *a. psychodynamic therapy.
   b. sex education.
   c. communication skills training.
   d. cognitive-behavioral therapy.

   Page: 585   Topic: Treatment

62. Treatment for sexual dysfunctions will likely include all of the following EXCEPT
   a. educating couples about sex.
   *b. a focus on the partner who is experiencing the problem.
   c. overcoming guilt about sexual needs and preferences.
   d. experimenting with masturbation to learn what gives pleasure.

   Page: 585   Topic: Treatment

63. Which of the following is NOT a sex myth?
   a. Men are always ready for sex.
   b. Sex should be spontaneous.
   *c. Women are aroused by erotic films and books.
   d. Menopause is the end of a woman's sex life.

   Page: 586   Topic: Highlight 13.7: Sex Myths

64. The technique that Masters and Johnson developed to help couples learn about the sex practices that give them pleasure is
   a. pause and squeeze
   b. the stuffing technique
   c. stop-start technique
   *d. sensate focus.

   Page: 585   Topic: Treatment

65. Xavier is being treated for premature ejaculation. He and his partner are likely to use which technique?
   *a. pause and squeeze
   b. the stuffing technique
   c. stop-start technique
   d. sensate focus

   Page: 586   Topic: Treatment

66. The story of jazz musician Billy Tipton demonstrates that
   a. women have to pretend they are men to succeed in certain occupations.
   *b. gender identity is a social and cultural construct that is only loosely related to biological facts.
   c. ultimately, even the most careful of transvestites will be found out.
   d. the boundaries between what constitutes a male and what constitutes a female, are very unclear.

   Pages: 588–589   Topic: Gender Identity Disorder

67. Howie never felt like a boy. Even though he was tall, he was thin and had beautifully fine, feminine features. He often dressed up in his sister's clothes, and his best friends were always girls with whom he would go shopping, play with dolls, go bike riding, and ice-skate. He often got beat up because he refused to fight back. In fact, he often refused to admit he was a boy because he thought they were so vulgar. Once he turned 18, Howie started therapy and ultimately had surgery to become a woman. This describes
    a. transvestism.
    b. homosexuality.
    *c. transsexualism.
    d. gender dysphoria.

    Page: 589   Topic: Description and Diagnosis

68. David is homosexual. This means
    a. he would like to be a female.
    b. he likes to dress in women's clothes.
    c. he has gender identity disorder.
    *d. he will likely experience prejudice.

    Page: 590   Topic: Critical Thinking About . . . 13.2: Changing the Sexual Orientation of Gay Men and Lesbians

69. The text cites the case of "John who became Joan" due to a surgical accident in which his penis was cut off at age 8 months. This case demonstrates that gender identification
    *a. is set before birth and cannot be changed by surgery or by social interaction.
    b. is not fixed at birth but rather is learned by social interaction.
    c. is not fixed at birth but rather can be altered through surgical intervention.
    d. is not yet sufficiently understood to identify what determines it.

    Page: 591   Topic: Etiology and Treatment

70. The condition known a pseudohermaphroditism suggests the notion that
    a. a person may be born with aspects of both female and male genitalia.
    *b. gender identity is determined more by the sex of a person's brain than by the appearance of their genitalia.
    c. gender identity is determined more by the appearance of a person's genitalia than by the sex of their brain.
    d. gender identity is determined more by a person's social interactions than by their brain or their genitalia.

    Page: 591   Topic: Etiology and Treatment

71. Research on people who have undergone a sex change operation finds that
    a. many wish to return to their original sex.
    b. a large number of them continue to have problems.
    *c. most are satisfied with the results of their sex-change operation.
    d. few are able to lead rewarding lives.

    Page: 592   Topic: Etiology and Treatment

TRUE-FALSE QUESTIONS

72. What constitutes acceptable sexual behavior is largely consistent around the world. (F)

    Page: 556   Topic: Paraphilias

73. During the 19th century in the United States, people risked jail for revealing desires such as masturbation. (T)

    Page: 556   Topic: Paraphilias

74. Von Krafft-Ebing believed that masturbation caused blindness. (F)

Page: 557   Topic: Paraphilias

75. The Internet is a new technology used for the very old purpose of searching for sex. (T)

Page: 560   Topic: Highlight 13.2: Surfing for Sex

76. Most rapes are committed by someone the victim does not know. (F)

Page: 562   Topic: Highlight 13.3: Rape Is Not Sex

77. Most paraphilias are not illegal. (T)

Page: 563   Topic: Paraphilias Not Otherwise Specified

78. High hormone levels have been found to cause paraphilias. (F)

Page: 567   Topic: Biological Causes

79. Once the paraphiliac's early experiences misdirect sexual impulses away from intimate social relationships and toward other sexual outlets, practically anything can take on sexual connotations. (T)

Page: 567   Topic: Social and Psychological Causes

80. At one time or another, practically everyone will have some problem performing a sex act. (T)

Page: 572   Topic: The Prey

81. Masters and Johnson found that there is considerable variability in the size of the erect penis. (F)

Page: 576   Topic: Human Sexual Response

82. Masters and Johnson showed that all female orgasms are caused by clitoral manipulation. (T)

Page: 576   Topic: Human Sexual Response

83. Generally speaking, multiple sexual dysfunctions are the exception rather than the rule. (F)

Page: 576   Topic: Human Sexual Response

84. Hypoactive sexual desire disorder rarely exists on its own. (T)

Page: 578   Topic: Sexual Desire Disorders

85. Sex addiction is defined as engaging in sex more than seven times a week with multiple sex partners. (F)

Page: 580   Topic: Highlight 13.6: Addicted to Sex

86. The term *erectile disorder* has replaced the term *impotence*. (T)

Page: 579   Topic: Sexual Arousal Disorders

87. Most women have pretty much the same needs with respect to the type and intensity of stimulation they require to achieve an orgasm. (F)

Page: 581   Topic: Orgasmic Disorders

88. It is possible for couples to have satisfying sex lives well into old age. (T)

Page: 582   Topic: Epidemiology and Course

89. Generally speaking, the popular media do a good job of disseminating accurate information about sexual dysfunctions. (F)

Page: 584   Topic: Treatment

90. The military's "don't ask, don't tell" policy is a way to provide homosexual members of the armed forces with the same civil rights that are available to heterosexual members. (F)

    Page: 590   Topic: Gay Men and Lesbians: An Ethical Quandary

91. It is unethical to change the sex of a person with a psychological disorder. (T)

    Pages: 591–592   Topic: Etiology and Treatment

SHORT-ANSWER QUESTIONS

92. Describe the characteristics of pedophiles.

    Most are males; they generally focus on children younger than age 13. Most are satisfied to fantasize about sex with children or to collect child pornography, but others act out their fantasies, usually with their own children or with children of friends or relatives. Some set out to meet children by becoming sports coaches, Big Brothers, or Scout leaders; a few prey on homeless children.

    Page: 556   Topic: The Predator

93. Describe the three intense sexual fantasies that characterize the paraphilias.

    sex with nonhuman objects (e.g., bras or panties); sex that involves suffering on the part of self or partner; sex with children

    Page: 558   Topic: Diagnosis

94. Describe the constitutional dilemma concerning sex and the Internet.

    The Internet is being used to procure children in sexual poses for pedophiles as well as to recruit young people to pose for such pictures and to engage in sex. The existence of pedophile sites on the Internet has caused many people to call for censorship and control. In a society that values free speech, the control of antisocial activities must be balanced with the protection of constitutional rights. Getting this balance correct is a major challenge facing legal authorities.

    Page: 560   Topic: Highlight 13.2: Surfing for Sex

95. Why is it so difficult to obtain accurate prevalence estimates for the paraphilias?

    First, people with paraphilias rarely seek clinical assistance. The meager prevalence figures come mainly from surveys of people convicted of sex crimes, who are not a representative sample of people with paraphilias because most paraphilias are not illegal. Second, paraphiliac behavior may be masked by other diagnoses, such as alcohol or drug intoxication or behavior related to a psychotic episode, and people with those behaviors would normally be diagnosed with substance intoxication or psychosis, respectively.

    Pages: 558–563   Topic: Diagnosis

96. Discuss the problems with research conclusions implicating hormone levels in the paraphilias.

    Most men with high hormone levels do not meet the diagnostic criteria for a paraphilia. Also, hormone levels are affected by various substances. Because people with paraphilias, especially those convicted of sex crimes, may also use substances, it is not clear whether higher-than-normal hormone levels are the cause of the paraphilias or the result of substance abuse.

    Page: 567   Topic: Biological Causes

97. Describe the three behavioral explanations for the development of paraphilias.

(1) Paraphiliacs can be classically conditioned, where, for example, women's clothing becomes the conditioned stimulus whose presence during masturbation leads to an association with the conditioned response of orgasm. (2) They can be operantly conditioned. For example, as a child, a person with transvestic fetishism may have been encouraged and rewarded for dressing as a female; over time, cross-dressing alone became a source of pleasure. (3) Modeling may play a role: Paraphiliac activity is common in pornography, and people without other sexual outlets may copy the behavior depicted in videos and magazines; once tried, this behavior may be reinforced by masturbation and orgasm.

Pages: 567–569   Topic: Social and Psychological Causes

98. Discuss two negative effects that pornographic materials are thought to have.

(1) They may provoke naive viewers into modeling unacceptable behaviors that, if reinforced through orgasm, may lead to the development of sexual disorders; and (2) they may stimulate people who already have antisocial sexual fantasies to act them out.

Page: 570   Topic: Treatment

99. Describe the physiological responses in the five phases of the sexual response cycle.

(1) Desire: the motivation to engage in sexual activity. (2) Excitement: begins with foreplay, which causes the secretion of sex hormones, increased heart rate and more rapid breathing, and blood flow to the genitals, causing them to swell. (3) Plateau: genitals continue to fill with blood; muscles tense; penis becomes erect, testes enlarge and are pulled up into the scrotum; clitoris retracts under its hood, and tissues of the vagina swell. (4) Orgasm: in females, strong genital sensations and warmth in the pelvic area followed by rhythmic muscle contractions; in males, the sensation of the ejaculate coming, followed by muscle contractions in the penis that propel semen through the urethra and out the urinary opening. (5) Resolution: gradual return of the body to its prior unstimulated condition; for men, there is a refractory period in which they are unable to have another orgasm.

Page: 576   Topic: Table 13.3: Five Phases of the Sexual Response Cycle

100. What disorders discussed in the text might accompany hypoactive sexual desire disorder?

Disturbances in the other phases of the sexual response cycle, especially in excitement or orgasm, frequently co-occur with hypoactive sexual desire disorder. Medical conditions, particularly those that cause pain during intercourse; various psychological disorders, such as depression or body dysmorphic disorder; and many drugs may also cause people to lose interest in sex.

Pages: 577–579   Topic: Sexual Desire Disorders

101. Discuss and give examples of the four primary reasons stated in the text for erectile dysfunction.

Aging: In general, older men need more stimulation and take longer to achieve an erection than do young men. Substances, such as anti-hypertensive drugs, alcohol, or tranquilizers. Medical disorders, such as diabetes or spinal jury. Other psychological disorders, such as depression, guilt, or performance anxiety.

Page: 579   Topic: Sexual Arousal Disorders

102. Discuss the three common factors that apply to treating most people with sexual dysfunction.

First, treatment is almost always focused on couples, even when one partner has the identified problem. Second, educating couples about sex is crucial: For example, women need to know that multiple orgasms are rare; men need to know that everyone experiences erectile failure sometimes. Third, couples need to overcome embarrassment and guilt about their sexual needs and preferences, and partners need to know what gives their lover pleasure and what does not.

Page: 585   Topic: Treatment

103. Describe Masters and Johnson's sensate focus technique.

Sensate focus helps couples learn about the sex practices that give them pleasure. It requires that one partner actively stimulate the other, who focuses on the pleasurable feelings being induced. The partners then switch roles, so that each takes a turn giving and receiving stimulation. Couples are encouraged to set aside time in quiet and relaxed settings. The active partner caresses the passive partner, giving pleasure but refraining from sexual intercourse. Treatment may begin by partners holding hands or giving back rubs. They gradually proceed to genital caresses and stimulation but do not proceed to intercourse until they can do so untroubled by performance anxiety. The idea is to concentrate on erotic sensations without the performance anxiety induced by the need to achieve orgasm.

Pages: 585–586   Topic: Treatment

104. Explain the start-stop technique for treating male erectile disorder.

It begins with the partner caressing the man until he gets an erection and then stopping. When the erection disappears, the partner repeats the caresses until the man is once again erect, and then stops. By repeating this start-stop cycle many times, the man gains confidence in his ability to achieve erections and learns that his erections occur naturally in response to stimulation.

Page: 586   Topic: Treatment

105. Describe the pause-and-squeeze treatment for premature ejaculation.

The male is stimulated until he signals that he feels orgasm coming. At that point, the partner stops the stimulation and squeezes the man's penis, which keeps the orgasmic process from being completed. As this "treatment" is repeated, ejaculation is gradually delayed. The couple then switches to vaginal stimulation in which brief periods of entry are followed by stopping until the male is able to engage in intercourse for a reasonable period of time without ejaculating.

Page: 586   Topic: Treatment

106. Explain the process for changing a person's sex.

Treatment usually begins by having the person live as the other gender for a trial period, during which time the person is carefully monitored for other psychological disorders. During the period, sex hormones are administered to produce many of the physical characteristics of the other sex—specifically, men are given estrogen, which causes them to develop breasts and makes their body and facial hair disappear, and women are given testosterone to deepen their voices, increase muscle mass, and cause body and facial hair to develop. Some people stop at this point. Others have sex-change surgery in which males are made to look like females and females are given artificial penises, which may be augmented with pumps or other erection-imitating mechanical devices to enable them to produce a sexual response.

Pages: 591–592   Topic: Etiology and Treatment

ESSAY QUESTIONS

107. As you come into your sociology class, you hear your classmates arguing loudly about the chapter they've just read on deviance. When they see you enter the room, they turn to you, as a psychology major, and ask you exactly how a psychologist determines that someone's sexual behavior is disordered. What could you tell them?

Here you will need to address the paraphilias, sexual dysfunctions, and gender identity disorder, paying primary attention to the distress that is caused to the person with the disorder and/or to others affected by it.

108. In a conversation with an old friend from grade school, you mention one of your best friends at college, who happens to be homosexual. Your old friend loses it, accusing you of "cavorting with those sinful, bestial creatures," and asking, "Don't you know what perverts they are! You should. You're the one who's studying sexual disorders!" Explain to your friend exactly what the different sexual disorders are and that homo-sexuality is *not* a sexual disorder.

    Describe the paraphilias, sexual dysfunctions, and gender identity disorder; then address the research on human sexuality generally and the wide range of normal human sexual activity, to set your friend "straight."

109. When you pick up the morning newspaper, this headline jumps out at you: JACK RIP, TWO-TIME CHILD RAPIST, RELEASED TODAY! As you read, you discover that after serving half the time to which he was sentenced, Mr. Rip is about to be released into your neighborhood. You are concerned because there are many young children living in your neighborhood. What issues are at stake here in terms of the danger to children, Mr. Rip's constitutional rights, and the law as it currently stands?

    You would discuss the likelihood that a sex offender will commit another sex crime, discuss Megan's Law and civil commitment, and balance those options against the sex offender's constitutional rights in terms of having served the sentence for the crime committed.

110. One of your cousins has confided in you that he and his wife are having some "problems with their intimacy." More specifically, he is unable to get an erection, and even if he could, his wife is "too small" to enter. He wants to know what they can do to "fix this" and have a satisfying sex life.

    Discuss the treatments for erectile disorder and vaginismus.

111. As you read this chapter on the sexual disorders, you wonder how life might be different for people who have one or more of these disorders—and how life might be different for the people who are affected or touched by these people. It seems clear that many people could avoid a great deal of suffering if we could find ways to prevent these disorders. Considering the etiology and course of sexual disorders, plan a prevention program.

    Here you need to discuss primary, secondary, and tertiary prevention for the paraphilias, the sexual dysfunctions, and gender identity disorder, plus an intervention to educate the public about accepting individual differences in sexual orientation—including homosexuality and transsexualism.

EPILOGUE:
LITTLETON, COLORADO, AND THE FUTURE
OF ABNORMAL PSYCHOLOGY

MULTIPLE-CHOICE QUESTIONS

1. As we enter the 21st century, _____ remains among the most debilitating of medical and psychological disorders.
    *a. schizophrenia
    b. bipolar disorder
    c. obsessive-compulsive disorder
    d. antisocial personality disorder

    Page: 596   Topic: Introduction

2. From reading the story of Eric Harris and Dylan Klebold, it would appear that
    a. they were "basically normal" teenagers.
    *b. many signs were overlooked that might have predicted their deadly actions.
    c. there were few signs, if any, that might have predicted their deadly actions.
    d. their counselors were concerned about the lack of progress they were making.

    Pages: 596–599   Topic: Normal Kids

3. With respect to their social interactions, at the time of their deadly shooting spree, Eric Harris and Dylan Klebold
    a. had managed to become members of the sports clique.
    b. belonged to the Trenchcoat Mafia.
    *c. were alienated from all the cliques at Columbine High.
    d. did not belong to any cliques but had several close friends in school.

    Pages: 598–600   Topics: Normal Kids; Unanswered Questions

4. According to the text, _____ one of the most important determinants of violent behavior.
    a   media violence is
    b. computer games are
    c. large schools are
    *d. peer influence is

    Page: 600   Topic: Unanswered Questions

5. Eric Harris was rejected by the Marine Corps because
    *a. he was taking Luvox (fluvoxamine).
    b. his high school grades were too low.
    c. he demonstrated poor behavior control.
    d. he had a criminal record.

    Pages: 600–601   Topic: How Do We Ensure . . . ?

6. Prescribing a drug for a condition other than the one for which it is FDA approved is
    a. illegal.
    *b. called off-label use.
    c. risky.
    d. uncommon.

    Page: 601   Topic: How Do We Ensure . . . ?

7. When clinicians use a therapeutic technique that has not previously been applied to a particular problem, they are
    a. being unethical.
    b. usually participating in a controlled study.
    *c. relying on their clinical judgment and intuition.
    d. doing a disservice to their clients.

    Page: 601   Topic: How Do We Ensure . . . ?

8. Dr. Mortorano is conducting a clinical trial of a treatment for schizophrenia. If he is using the typical protocol, we would expect him to select _____ as participants in his study.
    a. chronic schizophrenics
    b. a combination of chronic schizophrenics and nonschizophrenics
    c. a combination of chronic schizophrenics and those who are having their first episode of schizophrenia
    *d. people who are having their first episode of schizophrenia

    Page: 601   Topic: How Do We Ensure . . . ?

9. All of the following are likely to be problems when applying efficacious treatments in the real world of the clinic EXCEPT
    *a. type of clinical study.
    b. selecting clients who meet certain criteria.
    c. economics.
    d. clinician training.

    Page: 601   Topic: How Do We Ensure . . . ?

10. Currently, millions of people are suffering more than they should from schizophrenia because
    a. we don't yet have effective ways of treating those with this disorder.
    *b. the latest research findings are not being applied in practice.
    c. families have not been trained to deal effectively with members who have schizophrenia.
    d. the stigma attached to the disorder keeps those with schizophrenia from participating in society.

    Page: 602   Topic: How Do We Ensure . . . ?

11. A young person, such as Eric Harris, who uses the prescription drug Luvox (fluvoxamine) is most likely to
    a. have obsessive-compulsive disorder.
    b. have depression.
    *c. experience agitation.
    d. experience a psychotic episode.

    Page: 602   Topic: How Do We Ensure . . . ?

12. In the shooting tragedy at Columbine High School, the police considered pressing charges against the parents of Eric Harris and Dylan Klebold because
    a. the boys' actions apparently resulted from years of child abuse.
    b. parents are responsible for the actions of their children.
    c. they wanted to hold these parents up as an example of what happens when you let your children run amok.
    *d. the police were convinced that the Klebolds and the Harrises must have known of their sons' plans.

    Page: 602   Topic: Will the Biopsychosocial Model . . . ?

13. The text suggests that Dylan Klebold's interest in Nazism was related to all of the following EXCEPT
    *a. being subjected to years of early child abuse.
    b. displaced anger at his Jewish mother.
    c. a form of self-hate.
    d. the result of parental apathy or rejection.

    Page: 602   Topic: Will the Biopsychosocial Model . . . ?

14. The prevailing view today concerning child psychopathology is that _____ are the major determiners of behavior.
    a. parents
    *b. nature and peer pressure
    c. societal pressures
    d. drugs

    Page: 602   Topic: Will the Biopsychosocial Model . . . ?

15. According to Judith Rich Harris (1998), parents
    a. are the critical element in the development of a child's personality.
    b. and genetics play an equal role in the development of a child's personality.
    *c. have only a minimal long-term effect on the development of a child's personality.
    d. have less effect than genes, but more effect than children's peers, on the development of a child's personality.

    Pages: 602–603   Topic: Will the Biopsychosocial Model . . . ?

16. According to Judith Rich Harris (1998), a child's later behavior is affected by
    a. abusive parenting.
    b. neglect.
    c. early childhood experiences.
    *d. genetics.

    Page: 603   Topic: Will the Biopsychosocial Model . . . ?

17. The text notes that all of the following are signs of a society that has become pessimistic about its ability to improve the human condition EXCEPT
    *a. an emphasis on the importance of nurture on a child's development.
    b. habitual-criminal laws.
    c. the growing popularity of psychoactive drugs.
    d. the increasingly widespread belief that genes are the dominant force in behavior.

    Page: 603   Topic: Will the Biopsychosocial Model . . . ?

18. What belief has made possible the increased understanding of human behavior and improved quality of life for people with psychological disorders?
    a. A drug will eventually be found to cure, or at least to control, all abnormal behaviors.
    *b. Human behavior can be modified by environmental forces.
    c. Genetic therapy is the underlying key to changing unacceptable behaviors.
    d. A "gentler, kinder nation" will alleviate many social ills.

    Page: 604   Topic: Will the Biopsychosocial Model . . . ?

19. As pointed out in the text, the tragedy of Columbine High School underscores
    a. the necessity of ensuring that aggressive youngsters complete their diversion programs.
    b. that the sale of firearms and other weapons should be outlawed.
    *c. that psychologists are not very accurate at predicting rare violent events.
    d. the importance of strict parental supervision.

    Page: 604   Topic: How Do We Get Treatment and Prevention to Cooperate?

20. The text suggests that to help people like Eric Harris and Dylan Klebold, it is important to:
    a. provide extra counseling for troubled students.
    b. involve parents in their children's lives.
    c. develop school programs that teach children effective anger management strategies.
    *d. foster better cooperation across service providers.

    Page: 604   Topic: Will the Biopsychosocial Model . . . ?

21. The most common psychoactive drug prescribed for children is
    *a. Ritalin.
    b. Luvox.
    c. Haldol.
    d. Fen-phen.

    Page: 605   Topic: How Will Health Economics Affect Abnormal Psychology?

22. The majority of prescriptions for children and adolescents are written by
    a. psychiatrists.
    *b. family physicians.
    c. psychologists.
    d. physicians' assistants.

    Page: 605   Topic: How Will Health Economics Affect Abnormal Psychology?

23. Emily's parents take her to a family physician at their health maintenance organization to be treated for a behavior disorder. She will most likely receive
    a. a combination of drug therapy and psychological treatment.
    b. psychological treatment only.
    *c. drug treatment only.
    d. close monitoring of her behavior.

    Page: 605   Topic: How Will Health Economics Affect Abnormal Psychology?

24. The nation with the LEAST restrictive gun laws in the world, and one of the highest death rates from shootings, is
    a. Great Britain.
    b. Mexico.
    c. Italy.
    *d. the United States.

    Page: 605   Topic: Will Abnormal Psychology Have a Role . . . ?

25. The critical question for abnormal psychology to get society to understand concerning the relationship between the ease of acquiring guns and reducing violence is
    *a. "What are the cultural and psychological forces that glorify gun ownership?"
    b. "What are the constitutional issues to be resolved in limiting access to guns?"
    c. "How do we teach people to separate gun ownership from violence?"
    d. "How can we reduce access to deadly weapons"?

    Page: 605   Topic: Will Abnormal Psychology Have a Role . . . ?

26. According to the text, it would be important for Dr. Forward, a psychologist of the future, to focus on translating psychological discoveries into effective treatments for people who are treated in all of the following settings EXCEPT
   a. the clinic.
   *b. research.
   c. schools.
   d. the courts.

   Page: 606   Topic: The Way Forward

27. For the mental health of society, the text mentions the importance of progress in all of the following research domains EXCEPT
   a. basic research.
   b. treatment research.
   *c. educational research.
   d. services research.

   Page: 606   Topic: The Way Forward

28. Dr. Learned does research dealing with the mechanisms of learning and habit formation, how social forces influence behavior, and the importance of biological factors such as genetics. Dr. Learned is involved in _____ research.
   a. services
   b. treatment
   c. educational
   *d. basic

   Page: 606   Topic: Basic Research

29. Basic research has largely taken place within the context of which model of human behavior?
   *a. biopsychosocial
   b. biological
   c. psychoanalytic
   d. cognitive

   Page: 606   Topic: Basic Research

30. The text points out that _____ emerging as a primary source for making information about psychological disorders available worldwide.
   a. international conferences are
   *b. the Internet is
   c. teleconferencing is
   d. cooperation among scientists from different countries is

   Page: 606   Topic: Basic Research

31. As stated in the text, treatment research in the future will have to focus on all of the following EXCEPT
   a. lifelong studies.
   b. management strategies aimed at reducing relapses.
   *c. short-term outcomes with 2-year follow-ups.
   d. strategies aimed at providing those with mental disorders a high quality of life despite their disorders.

   Page: 606   Topic: Treatment Research

32. To collect information on clinical practice and outcomes _____ need to be developed.
    a. effective mental health treatment techniques
    b. cost-effective mental health treatment techniques
    c. sophisticated data analyses to study mental health care
    *d. measures of the quality of mental health care

    Page: 606   Topic: Treatment Research

33. Dr. Jones is concerned with the perennial problem of the long time lag between clinical research and its practical application. He has now learned that the way medical scientists get around this problem is by
    *a. forming data repositories in which the results of trials are collected.
    b. keeping in close communication with all other scientists conducting research in their field.
    c. hiring enough graduate students to keep up with the latest publications in the field.
    d. getting on all of the online e-mail lists that deal with their particular research interests.

    Page: 607   Topic: Treatment Research

34. Dr. Schwartz is concerned with the fragmented system that allows some people, like Eric Harris and Dylan Klebold, to "fall through the cracks." This concern relates to which research domain?
    a. basic
    *b. services
    c. treatment
    d. education

    Page: 607   Topic: Services Research

TRUE-FALSE QUESTIONS

35. For the first time in history, we are now able to treat the majority of mental disorders. (T)

    Page: 596   Topic: Introduction

36. Currently, depression is the leading cause of illness-related disability in the world. (F)

    Page: 596   Topic: Introduction

37. When Eric Harris and Dylan Klebold entered high school, they became increasingly isolated from other students. (T)

    Page: 598   Topic: Normal Kids

38. Exposure to violence in the media can turn nonmurderers into killers. (F)

    Page: 600   Topic: Unanswered Questions

39. Prescribing a drug for a condition other than the one for which it is FDA approved is both common and legal. (T)

    Page: 601   Topic: How Do We Ensure . . . ?

40. A treatment's effectiveness in the clinic is usually similar to its efficacy in a clinical trial. (F)

    Page: 601   Topic: How Do We Ensure . . . ?

41. Psychologists are more likely to measure treatment efficacy than to measure treatment effectiveness. (T)

    Page: 601   Topic: How Do We Ensure . . . ?

42. It may be safely assumed from the off-label prescription use of Luvox (fluvoxamine) by Eric Harris that he suffered from depression. (F)

    Page: 602   Topic: How Do We Ensure . . . ?

43. Contrary to earlier beliefs, people working in the field of abnormal psychology today assume that the parents are to blame for their children's misbehavior. (F)

    Page: 602   Topic: Will the Biopsychosocial Model . . . ?

44. According to Judith Rich Harris (1998), parental influence is a stronger determinant of a child's behavior than peer influence is. (F)

    Page: 603   Topic: Will the Biopsychosocial Model . . . ?

45. A critical element in helping troubled kids like Eric Harris and Dylan Klebold is to foster better cooperation across service providers. (T)

    Page: 604   Topic: How Do We Get Treatment . . . ?

46. The most common drug prescribed for children today is Ritalin. (T)

    Page: 604   Topic: How Do We Get Treatment . . . ?

47. The majority of prescriptions for children are written by psychiatrists. (F)

    Page: 604   Topic: How Do We Get Treatment . . . ?

48. The United States has the LEAST restrictive gun laws in the world. (T)

    Page: 605   Topic: Will Abnormal Psychology . . . ?

49. If abnormal psychology is to have a practical effect on reducing violence, it must help society understand why we glorify gun ownership. (T)

    Page: 605   Topic: Will Abnormal Psychology . . . ?

50. The most important of the research domains for advancing the progress of the mental health of society is the basic research domain. (F)

    Page: 606   Topic: The Way Forward

51. To avoid incidents such as the tragedy at Columbine High School, the most critical aspect of human behavior to understand is the biological. (F)

    Page: 606   Topic: The Way Forward

52. The development of treatment guidelines to help clinicians decide which treatment to recommend next when the first is unsuccessful will lead to a discontinuation of "off-label" treatments. (F)

    Pages: 606–607   Topic: Treatment Research

53. It is important for clinicians to know more about how services are actually provided to clients. (T)

    Page: 607   Topic: Services Research

54. Even the best treatments will not produce good outcomes if the systems for implementing them fail to work. (T)

    Page: 607   Topic: Services Research

SHORT-ANSWER QUESTIONS

55. What type of high school experience did Eric Harris and Dylan Klebold have that might have led to the tragedy at Columbine High School?

    When they entered high school, they became increasingly isolated from other students. They tried to join a school clique whose distinctive form of dress earned it the name Trenchcoat Mafia, but even this "alternative" group rejected them. The two boys wore long coats but never made it past the periphery of that clique. Harris began to call himself Reb, and he began to show a tendency toward melodrama. His homecoming date refused to go out with him again, so he staged a fake suicide complete with imitation blood. By their junior year, Harris and Klebold no longer appeared clean-cut, they often spoke German, and they glorified Nazis. Their appearance and behavior made them a target for bullying; members of the football team abused them, called them names, and jostled them in the corridors.

Pages: 598–599   Topic: Normal Kids

56.   What are the two sides of the argument concerning the banning of violent computer games and music with violent lyrics to reduce the occurrence of violent behavior?

By limiting freedom of speech, we may reduce the risk of violence, but not by much. Exposure to violence in the media, or even in real life, does not, by itself, turn a nonmurderer into a killer. Temperament and peer influences are more important determinants of violent behavior than media violence. There may be more justification in calls to censor the Internet. However, because censorship pits freedom of speech against the potentially greater need for public safety, the topic will be debated for a long time.

Page: 600   Topic: Unanswered Questions

57.   Describe the procedures used in a controlled clinical trial.

In controlled clinical trials, clients are carefully selected to be as similar to one another as possible, with great pains taken to rule out extraneous factors. Participants are randomly assigned to treatment and control conditions. Participating clinicians are carefully trained in the treatment protocol and, where possible, are also kept "blind." Therapeutic regimens and processes are carefully specified so that all participants receive exactly the same treatment. By following these procedures, scientists can use statistical methods to measure a treatment's efficacy.

Pages: 601–602   Topic: How Do We Ensure. . . ?

58.   Describe the change that has taken place in the prevailing view of the development of child psychopathology.

Earlier in the century, those working in the field of abnormal psychology would have assumed that the parents were somehow to blame. Currently, parental nurture has given way to nature and peer pressure as the major determiners of behavior.

Pages: 602–604   Topic: Will the Biopsychosocial Model . . . ?

59.   What are the three signs the text discusses that indicate that society has become pessimistic about its ability to improve the human condition?

Habitual criminal laws, the growing popularity of psychoactive drugs, and the increasingly widespread belief that genes are the dominant force in our behavior.

Page: 603   Topic: Will the Biopsychosocial Model . . . ?

60.   What two steps does the text suggest those in the field of abnormal psychology use to confront the realities of managed care?

Research the patterns of care that people receive and formulate treatment guidelines to help family physicians improve the quality of the services they offer to people with mental disorders.

Page: 605   Topic: How Will Health Economics . . . ?

61.   What are the three interacting research domains stated in the text that are critical for the mental health of society?

basic research, treatment research, services research

Page: 606   Topic: The Way Forward

ESSAY QUESTIONS

62. Your cousin knows you have been taking this class in abnormal psychology and says to you, "You know, nothing has really changed in that field since the days of Freud. Why are you wasting your time?" What could you tell him about the current state of abnormal psychology?

    Discuss the biological, behavioral, and psychological advances that have occurred over the past 100 years.

63. You have been asked to address a local parents' group about the future of abnormal psychology and where the field is headed. They have specifically asked you to address the question "As we enter the new millennium, what are the most important questions facing abnormal psychology?" What could you tell them?

    Address the unanswered questions, such as how we ensure that scientific findings work in the clinic, whether the biopsychosocial model will survive, etc.

64. Your advisor is conducting a forum on the future of psychology and its role in improving society in the next millennium. You have been asked to address the question "How should abnormal psychology evolve to ensure that it meets its goals of understanding, treating, and preventing mental disorders?" What could you tell your audience?

    Address the important interaction of basic research, treatment research, and services research; also address the issues of cooperation/communication/collaboration and economics.